The
Endometriosis
Answer Book:
New Hope, New Help

Other Books by Niels H. Lauersen, M.D., Ph.D.

Childbirth with Love

It's Your Body (with Steven Whitney)

It's Your Pregnancy

Listen to Your Body (with Eileen Stukane)

PMS: Premenstrual Syndrome and You (with Eileen Stukane)

The
Endometriosis
Answer Book:
New Hope, New Help

Niels H. Lauersen, M.D., Ph.D.,
and Constance deSwaan

FAWCETT COLUMBINE • NEW YORK

A Fawcett Columbine Book
Published by Ballantine Books

Copyright © 1988 by Niels H. Lauersen and Constance deSwaan

Library of Congress Catalog Card Number: 88-92041

ISBN: 0-449-90361-3

This edition published by arrangement with Rawson Associates, a division of Macmillan Publishing Company.

Cover design by Sheryl Kagan

Manufactured in the United States of America

First Ballantine Books Edition: April 1989
10 9

To the future good health of all women with endometriosis.
May our combined knowledge and efforts
help eliminate this problem.

Contents

Acknowledgments

Patients, colleagues, and friends—men and women both—have encouraged me to write a comprehensive guide about pelvic endometriosis for any woman who is confused or curious about the symptoms, prevention, and best medical recommendations for treatment and cure of this disease. *The Endometriosis Answer Book* is the result. I hope it will provide the answers to their many often-asked questions about the management of endometriosis and what *they* can do to fight it.

Many of these people contributed in some way to this book, and my deepest gratitude goes to each of them:

The collection of research materials was done by Dr. Yanni Antonopoulos, Donna Brummett, Joanne Cardillo, Tom Giordano, Rachelle Goldman, Margola Gross, Lori Leeds, Leigh Shearin, Maxine Siegler, and Kathleen H. Wilson. Their assistance, comments, and perceptions are profoundly appreciated.

The original artwork was done by Laurel Purington Rand. I also want to thank Adrian Rothenberg and Tom Saltarelli for their graphic art.

Special thanks also go to the nurses and assistants in my office, especially Joan Affigne, Paula Friedman, Louisa Giannattasio, and Kristen McLeod, who have generously helped patients and sufferers of this disease.

My appreciation also extends to many others who have aided in the preparation of this book: Deborah Alessi, Emily Altman, Carolyn Bloom, Michelle DeLuca, Barbara Fila, Deborah Goldstein, Karen Gray, Linda Greenberg, Judy Gregory, Barbara Grover, Kathy Hughes-Morris, Joni Ives, Lori Johnson, Jacqueline Krasnoff, Adele Kreji, Bill Kreji, Lynette Long, Barbara Morris, Lynn Paige, Joe Policano, Denise Rice, Joan Rongione, Jennifer Rouse, Michelle Szackacs, Channie Tolchinski, Carol Torrisi, and Marsha Winkler.

Thanks to Mary Ann Schoudel, who transcribed some tapes for us.

My good wishes go to all my patients and the many women with endometriosis who have consulted with me or written to me about their own experience with the disease. Their stories, which form the basis of this guide, have given it an invaluable authenticity.

Special thanks go to my colleagues—physicians throughout the country who have been instrumental in battling endometriosis: Dr. J. Victor Reyniak, Dr. Robert Greenblatt, Dr. Robert Kistner, Dr. Fritz Fuchs, Dr. Paul Dmowski, Dr. John Stangel, Dr. Donald Chatman, Dr. Veasy Buttram, Dr. Robert Geller, Dr. John Rock, Dr. Gerson Weiss, Dr. Robert Atkins, Dr. Christiane Northrup, and Dr. Ronald Hoffman. Special thanks to Dr. Patricia Conrad, for her valuable assessment of the manuscript.

My appreciation goes to psychologists Rona Silverton and Dr. Fern Kaslow and to acupuncturist/herbalist Abigail Rist, for their insights into women's health care.

Special acknowledgment goes to Mary Lou Ballweg, founder and executive director of the Endometriosis Society. Ms. Ballweg and I years ago shared the position of explaining on television an insidious problem newly on the rise, endometriosis, and why it must be stopped as soon as possible. Her efforts have done much to increase the awareness and prevention of the disease.

Many thanks to Alice Martell, my agent, for her support during the preparation of this manuscript.

My appreciation to my legal advisor, Richard Allen, for his interest and advice on this project.

Finally, my gratitude goes to my publisher and editor, Eleanor Rawson, and editor in chief, Toni Sciarra, for their wisdom, patience, and guidance in producing this book.

Niels H. Lauersen, M.D.
New York, 1987

To the editors of this book, without whom this opportunity would have been impossible.

To Harris Diamant and to the Wednesday Night Writers' Group— Lauri Peters, Mary Bringle, Patricia Mullen, Kathryn Marx, Mary Lou Moore, and Gay-Darlene Bidart—without whom I would have been impossible.

And to Marie-Louise Grish and Xomalin Peralta, for their unfailing good humor and support.

Constance deSwaan
New York, 1987

SPECIAL NOTE:

Except for the women physicians or other women experts who are specifically quoted in this book, we have used the male pronouns *he, him,* and *his* when referring to hypothetical or unnamed doctors. Such identifying usage is meant only to distinguish the woman patient (referred to as *she, her,* and *hers*) from her gynecologist or other health care professional. The description of the doctor as male and the patient as female carries with it no political or personal opinions about the capabilities of either male or female physicians or other practitioners.

N.H.L. and C.deS., April 1987

The
Endometriosis
Answer Book:
New Hope, New Help

CHAPTER 1

Endometriosis: The Good News

WILL I ever feel normal again?"

Charlotte asked the question, then lowered her eyes. She seemed embarrassed, as if she'd brought up a dismal subject when pleasantries were more in order. As she sat opposite me that morning, I knew she was thinking in terms of bad news, not cure.

The irony was that Charlotte's question was perfectly appropriate for the situation. I was her doctor and she'd come to my office to be examined for problems that had long been troubling her. Charlotte had been suffering from various forms of abdominal discomfort and severe pelvic pain. For years, no doctor had been able to help her or tell her what was wrong. Lately, she'd begun to personalize the pain, blaming herself for it. "What other reason *is* there?" she asked in despair.

Although we'd met before today, Charlotte was a new patient. She had come for a third opinion on her condition and she was clearly worried about my diagnosis. I had seen Charlotte in the hospital's neonatal nursery, where she worked as a pediatrics nurse specializing in the care of premature infants. I knew her there as a capable, responsible professional and a self-proclaimed perfectionist. At this moment, however, she was beset by shyness, vulnerable and frightened.

"I believe you have endometriosis," I finally told her, "but I feel we're catching it early enough for a complete cure."

The news brought a flush to her face. "I had a suspicion that it *was* endometriosis," she said, "and in a strange way, I'm relieved. At least I know the suffering I have been going through is from a real disease." She paused and looked at me intently. "Tell me the truth—do you think I'll ever be able to have a child?"

Charlotte feared that putting off childbirth until her thirties might have a tragic consequence for her: sterility. It is a bitter reality. Charlotte knew that infertility affected thousands of working women. She suspected that conception would be additionally difficult because of her last few years of chronic pain.

"Yes, I'm almost certain you can have children," I assured her, "but first we must get the endometriosis under control and your general health back on track. It is possible that you will need specific fertility treatments later on," I continued, "but we'll deal with that as it comes up. Most of all, and most important for you, I believe we caught the disease in time!"

THERE IS HOPE

What Charlotte is facing at this time in her life is not unique to her. Millions of other women are also suffering from endometriosis, and many of them don't know they have the disease. Charlotte, in one sense, was lucky. Since she is a nurse and has medical knowledge, she was aware of what the symptoms could mean.

The two gynecologists whom she had consulted over the last few years held similar opinions, stated in different terms. The first one repeatedly told her she was just suffering from bad menstrual cramps. Eventually, his lack of interest in her case led Charlotte to seek a second specialist. He, too, blamed her pain on menstrual cramps *and* the effects of excessive work-related tension. When she suggested that endometriosis might be the cause, he told her she was being overly dramatic.

Charlotte began to doubt herself. Maybe her problem *was* just menstrual cramps. She brought up the subject one night after dinner with two of her women friends—what did they think? Both of them advised her wisely: get another opinion from a doctor who specializes in treating endometriosis. She was given a few names to call, and mine was among them. Armed with some knowledge and an inner conviction that she was suffering from a *real* disease, Charlotte made an appointment to see me.

When I heard the heartbreaking details of Charlotte's solitary battle with endometriosis, I realized that her story, and others like it, must be told. Charlotte, in many ways, shares a common medical history with an enormous number of women; she is suffering and in pain, yet doctors have misdiagnosed her problem. What matters most is that she did not give up in her search for treatment and cure.

This book is for Charlotte and all women like her who are suffering and who have endometriosis, whether they are aware of their disease or not. The knowledge, support, and motivation to seek help found within these pages will be your first weapon toward combating this insidious disease. As a gynecologist and obstetrician specializing in treating this disorder, I am confident that there is hope! What matters is early detection. If the disease is caught early enough, the cure rate can almost be an astounding 100 percent. With the right doctor and the material presented in this book, you will learn how to prevent the onset of the disease. If you are a sufferer, you can ease your pain and prevent its recurrence.

I have seen thousands of women with endometriosis at every stage. I have listened to women talk about their symptoms—and I have been angry on learning that they had often been misdiagnosed and then treated over long periods of time for conditions they did not have. I sympathize with the pain they feel, and the sense of confusion they may experience when asking: *Why me? How did I get this disease?*

In the many national television appearances I have made, the subject of endometriosis generates enthusiastic response and dozens of questions from the studio audience. Thousands of letters reach me each year from women who have read my books, which include *It's Your Body, Listen to Your Body, PMS: Premenstrual Syndrome and You,* and *Childbirth with Love.* Nearly 70 percent of these letters focus on the trials of endometriosis. Sometimes they describe extremes of loss: cases of women in their early twenties who have been "cured" with hysterectomies. Other letters exult at the triumphs: women in their early forties who have been mercifully and knowledgeably cured, and now have a new baby!

My purpose as a caring doctor is to direct women toward their own triumphs of good health. For me, this means ending the suffering of endometriosis—the single greatest goal in my writing a book such as this. Realistically, I know I cannot combat this disease alone. I want to motivate women toward being active, knowledgeable partners in their own health care. Do as Charlotte did: find a specialist if you suspect that you might have endometriosis. (I'll explore how to begin your search for a doctor in the next chapter.)

After reading this book, you will know what physical signals to look for (including *pain*—where it occurs and at what frequency) and how to be aware of the subtle hormonal changes in your body that could mean early detection of this disease. You will learn what questions to ask your doctor and how to keep a diary of symptoms, including when they are most bothersome. I would like to make you a co-worker with your doctor in fighting this disease, using your knowledge and his to excise endometriosis from your life.

There is hope.

ENDOMETRIOSIS UP CLOSE: COULD YOU HAVE IT?

Let me briefly explain what endometriosis is and what happened to Charlotte. Endometriosis is inextricably linked to the simplest female biological function: menstruation. Every month, if there is no conception, endometrial cells lining the uterus slough off and exit the

THE MENSTRUAL CYCLE

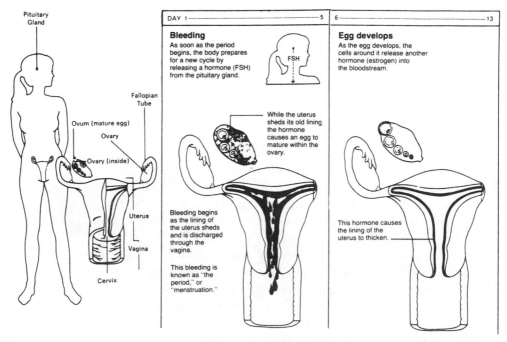

Pituitary Gland

Fallopian Tube

Ovum (mature egg)

Ovary

Ovary (inside)

Uterus

Vagina

Cervix

DAY 1 —————————— 5   6 ———————————— 13

Bleeding
As soon as the period begins, the body prepares for a new cycle by releasing a hormone (FSH) from the pituitary gland.

FSH

While the uterus sheds its old lining, the hormone causes an egg to mature within the ovary.

Bleeding begins as the lining of the uterus sheds and is discharged through the vagina.

This bleeding is known as "the period," or "menstruation."

Egg develops
As the egg develops, the cells around it release another hormone (estrogen) into the bloodstream.

This hormone causes the lining of the uterus to thicken.

4

body as menstrual blood. (See illustration.) When endometriosis takes hold, it is because of an abnormal "backing up" of these cells through the fallopian tubes. They "run wild," and under certain conditions they will *implant themselves* on abdominal organs. If the implants stick, they can cause extreme pain. As they grow, spread, and go undetected and untreated, they can cause, among other problems, cysts, tumors, and irreversible sterility.

This is a disease that is somewhat shrouded in mystery. No one yet knows its absolute cause or why it claims the victims it does. It is also a disease that can go undetected or misdiagnosed. Charlotte is a testimony to this all-too-common medical mistake. Why? Endometriosis tends to show itself first as severe menstrual cramps. Often, as a result of the growing implanted endometrial cells, it may form into ovarian tumors or cause symptoms that masquerade as a bladder infection. This is just the beginning.

What happens then? Charlotte, for one, told me that she'd suddenly begun suffering from menstrual cramps about three years before, at the age of twenty-four. This struck her as odd, since she was free of most premenstrual symptoms throughout her teenage years. Then, one night, she doubled over with what she thought, at first, was an appendix attack. Cramps this severe were not unusual for her from

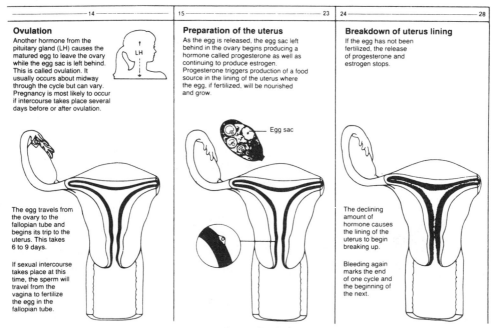

| 14 | 15 | 23 | 24 | 28 |

Ovulation

Another hormone from the pituitary gland (LH) causes the matured egg to leave the ovary while the egg sac is left behind. This is called ovulation. It usually occurs about midway through the cycle but can vary. Pregnancy is most likely to occur if intercourse takes place several days before or after ovulation.

The egg travels from the ovary to the fallopian tube and begins its trip to the uterus. This takes 6 to 9 days.

If sexual intercourse takes place at this time, the sperm will travel from the vagina to fertilize the egg in the fallopian tube.

Preparation of the uterus

As the egg is released, the egg sac left behind in the ovary begins producing a hormone called progesterone as well as continuing to produce estrogen. Progesterone triggers production of a food source in the lining of the uterus where the egg, if fertilized, will be nourished and grow.

Egg sac

Breakdown of uterus lining

If the egg has not been fertilized, the release of progesterone and estrogen stops.

The declining amount of hormone causes the lining of the uterus to begin breaking up.

Bleeding again marks the end of one cycle and the beginning of the next.

Used with permission of the Syntex Corporation, Palo Alto, CA

5

then on. Three years later, she had become an aficionado, as she called it, of over-the-counter as well as prescription painkillers. She was close to being addicted when her boyfriend insisted she find help as soon as possible.

Charlotte's doctor told her that her menstrual cramps were hormone-related; she was made to feel that it was her misfortune to have whatever imbalance made them a wrenching nightmare a few days every month. A second doctor, upon a routine examination, suggested high-dosage birth control pills to ease the menstrual cramps. The pills helped for a few months, then lost their effectiveness. A year before she came to me, the doctor found a cyst on one of her ovaries and prescribed a drug to shrink it. When the drug didn't work, he suggested another. Through this, no one but her boyfriend knew of her suffering. To the world, she was Charlotte, the efficient professional, a very well-liked and often envied woman—someone you would want as a friend, someone always upbeat and on your side.

It was a concerned friend of hers at the hospital nursery who insisted that Charlotte call me. By the time she came for a consultation, the pelvic pain had become severely debilitating, and it was interfering with her work. What troubled her most and kept her postponing a visit to me was the fear of hearing the worst—that she would need an ovary removed or, worse, a hysterectomy. Such verdicts from a doctor are devastating to a young woman who has not yet had her family.

She wisely put her reservations aside and made the appointment to come to my office. There, I was able to correctly diagnose and subsequently treat her condition. What I thought best for her case was Danocrine, an antihormone that stops menstruation and gives pelvic organs a rest. (You will learn all about the pros and cons of all known treatments, including drugs such as Danocrine, and even alternative medicine, later on in this book.) Along with this drug, I recommended a special diet I have devised that cuts down on foods that affect hormone levels and cystic growth (more on this, too, in a later chapter). Most important, Charlotte had a chance to control and cure her endometriosis. The same is possible for you!

WOMEN, WORK, AND ENDOMETRIOSIS: UNCOVERING THE LINK

You may have something in common with Charlotte other than the physical symptoms of the disease. You may be a striving, working woman in your twenties or thirties who has put off childbearing to pursue a career. In another profile, you may be a woman of approximately Charlotte's age with one or two young children, and you, too, live a high-stress life, working and caring for a family. A surprising third portrait reveals you as a teenage girl, highly sensitive, but with a strong sense of competition that may or may not be fully expressed.

What do personal issues of fulfillment through work, or work as a matter of sheer economic survival, have to do with endometriosis? Don't *unambitious*, *nonstriving* women—even altruistic, spiritual women—develop the disease? Certainly they do! But they are not the most vulnerable. *In these transitional times, working women are most likely to succumb to endometriosis.*

How do I know this?

I'm a gynecologist, a specialist in women's health issues, a scientist who weighs and measures the minutiae of laboratory research before making an informed decision, but I am also a pragmatist and a humanitarian. I see who suffers from what and I set about to help them in an efficient and compassionate manner. And so I notice that nearly 95 percent of endometriosis patients are women under extreme stress who work or who have worked.

I know this is true because I treat these women every day and observe how they suffer the most pernicious consequences of endometriosis. In the 1980s it is nearly impossible for a gynecologist and obstetrician to care sensibly for a patient without identifying, describing, and fully examining some crucial details of her personal life. As part of treating the *person*, not just the symptoms, we must examine the external influences—physiological and psychological—that create changes in her health.

These are exciting times for women with professional aspirations, with greater chances than ever for taking on new responsibilities. In 1985, one-third of American earning power was a result of women's work on every level. In 1970, 26 percent of women between eighteen and twenty-four years of age were unmarried. In 1986, *56 percent* of the same age group were single—most of them in the work force. More relevant to our story, in 1950, 80 percent of women had borne at least one child by the age of thirty, whereas today, the figure has dropped to 60 percent.

Beyond job stress, women are juggling the minute-to-minute priorities of work and intimacy, confronting any ambivalence about achievement along with conflicts over dependency on men, figuring out how to achieve a *balance* on a day-to-day basis—and they are postponing childbirth.

Endometriosis isn't fair. It isn't interested in how hard a woman works and it doesn't care why a woman has not had children early in life, when there are fewer chances of organic complications. It thrives on stress-related immune system weakness, which, along with other factors that I will discuss in great detail later on, can control a woman's body and her life. But it needn't happen this way. *With my plan, you can learn to control endometriosis* and not feel that you must choose between your work and your health.

Describing endometriosis as the "career woman's" or working woman's disease may be the switch that turns on a highly charged debate among doctors, scientists, and even victims of the disease. But whatever else may be so, the change in life-style is here to stay, and it is every women's right to pursue the optimal health she desires in order to live a fully productive life.

CHAPTER 2

Finding the Right Doctor for You

ALTHOUGH we wish him to be heroic, loving, compassionate, wise, available to us at any time of day, fascinated by our particular case, skilled in matters of medicine as well as accomplished in the subtle manners of handling people, brilliant diagnosticians, chatty, charitable, and good-humored, we may find we are on a quest for the doctor who only *rarely* exists, if at all. We want a doctor who is a good person and a caring practitioner, but we may also be asking for him to be a god.

Many doctors incline toward a role as a lesser god. This can cause some conflict between such doctors and the patient who is a reluctant worshiper. Doctors who live the god role may be exemplary diagnosticians, dazzling surgeons, insightful theoreticians, awesome innovators—but they may not be able to talk simply, directly, and kindly to a patient. With a deep need to be sure of themselves, they can dismiss a patient who asks questions that require more information or explanation. Women doctors are not exempt from the god complex, even though we somehow expect them or wish them to be.

Most of us doctors are vitally connected to the needs of our patients. We know that we cannot make an accurate diagnosis unless we listen to the patient. We are aware of the advances in our particular field and apply them when it is possible. Although every doctor is different, his diagnostic skill, compassion, and general knowledge will depend on his social personality and inner disposition, his general sensitivity and training in his field.

My personal philosophy is simple: every patient is an individual and must be treated individually. At the same time, a woman must understand what is wrong with her, how she might have gotten a disorder, what she can do to cure it and prevent recurrence, and what I must do to make her well. With a disease like endometriosis, it is critical for doctors to listen carefully to symptoms and to medical histories. My fear is that too many women go undiagnosed when the disease is in its early stage, making it possible for the disease later to spread out of control.

My years as a gynecologist have shown that the most effective method of deciding if a doctor is right for you is if you can say *yes* to the following statements after discussing your case with him.

1. **Is my doctor a partner in my health care?** This is *the* critical question to ask yourself after first consulting with a doctor. Do you feel as if he cares about you? Or do you get the distinct impression that he expects you to do as he suggests, without question, including options for surgery?

2. **Can I talk openly about my medical problems with my doctor?** You should feel an immediate rapport with your doctor so that you are not intimidated into silence, thereby omitting what can be essential information to treating your case. If you cannot speak freely with your doctor, you are doing yourself a disservice. Find another with the right chemistry for you.

3. **Do I feel confidence in my doctor's ability?** You must feel that your doctor understands your condition and know that he is willing to explain it to you. Can he correctly diagnose and treat your problem so that it does not become worse over time? If you are seeing a doctor who repeatedly tells you that your symptoms are psychosomatic—when *you* know you are suffering from real pain—he may be missing the diagnosis. If you feel lagging confidence in your doctor, remember that *you are entitled to a second opinion.* Do not worry what the first doctor will think about this if he finds out. It is your body, your health, and your right to seek the best medical care.

4. **Do I feel safe knowing that my doctor doesn't rush into the more radical approaches to treatment?** Among the most common complaints against doctors are the rash use of prescription drugs and unnecessary surgery. Endometriosis sufferers tend to be suscepti-

ble to such mistreatments. In my experience, I have seen or corresponded with too many women who have agreed to costly surgery that they did not need. If your doctor appears eager to operate, suggesting that he will "save everything" he can, immediately seek a second opinion and, if necessary, a third or fourth. *You* want to save everything you can, too: your internal organs. And if you are taking prescription drugs that have ill effects or no effect, or if you think you are becoming addicted to a drug, tell your doctor. If he insists that you continue on the drug and dismisses your discomfort, find another doctor.

These are the key factors in selecting the right doctor. If after evaluating your answers, it is strikingly clear that you need a different specialist, be assured that you are not alone. Other women with endometriosis have had similar experiences. Fortunately, such women can be found, and they *communicate!* How? One avenue of communication, among others like it, is the pioneering Endometriosis Association, based in Milwaukee (with some branches in other cities), which can help guide women toward a doctor in or near their home area. In the appendix, I reveal how to plug into a vast network of support groups and supply further guidance on how to find a specialist in endometriosis who is right for you.

How I Became Interested in Curing Women of Endometriosis

I was a medical student at the University of Copenhagen in Denmark, my native country, when I felt an inclination toward specializing in obstetrics and gynecology. My choice was sealed when I accepted a chance to complete my fourth year of study at other European medical schools. This extraordinary year gave me the opportunity to observe how other cultures—French, Italian, German, British, Greek, and Swedish—manage disease and treat patients.

It was in Sweden that I witnessed the case of endometriosis that had a lasting impression on me.

I was studying with one of the professors at the Karolinska Institute in Stockholm, observing him as he saw his patients. Late one day, a lovely married woman in her late twenties arrived at his office, looking distraught. Her complaint was that she could not conceive after two years of trying. She had never been pregnant, even though she had been recklessly blithe about birth control on occasion. Another symptom was severe menstrual cramps.

11

This was the mid-1960s and the issue on many women's minds was how to *prevent* pregnancy, not how to achieve it. (Remember, this was before oral contraceptives or intrauterine devices became popular and legally accessible. Many women feared unwanted pregnancy and worried about the consequences of illegal abortions.) Here was a woman with the opposite problem.

This doctor was an exceptionally astute diagnostician. Even before examining her, he said that she was a victim of endometriosis. I began asking questions, wondering what her chances were to become fertile. The irony is that twenty-five years ago, doctors often recommended pregnancy as a *cure* for endometriosis, since pregnancy gives the body nine months of rest from disturbing menstrual periods. But how can you recommend pregnancy to a woman who is infertile? For her, surgery to clear away some of the implants appeared to be her only chance for motherhood.

I came to America to finish my training and conduct my internship at New York Hospital–Cornell Medical Center in New York City. There, I continued my education and training as a resident in obstetrics and gynecology. It was during my training in 1968 that a historic advance was made that would help endometriosis victims: a team of Swedish doctors perfected the laparoscope, an instrument with a narrow, drinking straw–shaped needle. This ingenious instrument revolutionized the diagnosis of endometriosis.

Simply explained, the laparoscope is inserted into the abdomen, allowing doctors to see into the pelvic cavity *without the need for major surgery*. Locating signs of endometriosis is therefore much easier.

This Swedish team introduced the laparoscope to American doctors and to surgical tool manufacturers. When they arranged to train several groups of doctors in the use of this instrument, I had the opportunity to study the technique firsthand with them. Following this, the first medical papers were published in the United States on laparoscopy (the technique named for the use of the tool), thereby making the process known and available to every doctor around the world. Laparoscopy still provides clinicians and researchers a valuable diagnostic tool often needed for the discovery of and ongoing research into endometriosis.

Early in my training, and when I opened my own practice, I was saddened by stories of how women were treated inhumanely by overworked or underinterested emergency room doctors and even by their own gynecologists. These were women in pain, being damned as carriers of venereal disease, or called overwrought from premenstrual hormone fluctuations. Why? Because some symptoms of endo-metriosis can mirror advanced stages of other disorders.

Over the years, my work with endometriosis patients intensified as women's life-styles changed and complaints of infertility were becom-ing more common. I have participated in many studies on various drug and treatment modes. I have written papers for medical journals and I feel sure that I have spoken more on the importance of early diagnosis of endometriosis even without laparoscopy or surgery than any other American doctor. I have cured thousands of women and I know there is an answer for *you* in this book.

WHAT THIS BOOK WILL REVEAL TO YOU

I want to share my knowledge of endometriosis in all its forms and stages, and demystify it for you. We'll start with the basics—what endometriosis is and what it can look like. If you're a sufferer—or if you have a relative or friend with the problem—chapters 3 and 4 will describe the ailment as you know it, from the earliest symptoms to the extremes of pain and even the confusion and the problems involved when doctors either misdiagnose the disorder or deny that it exists. These chapters will tell you how the disease can masquerade as an-other disorder and what doctors know about *how* endometriosis takes hold. To learn *why* endometriosis happens (discovering the actual causes are still more problematic than understanding *how* the disease manifests itself), read about the usually acknowledged theories in chapter 5.

I fervently believe that doctors must be partners in a patient's health care, but the advantage is on the side of the doctor unless the patient is educated about her condition and knows what to ask. Chapter 6 will teach you about the symptomology and diagnosis of the disease, along with providing a series of questions to ask of doctors.

Chapters 7 through 11 explore medical treatments, diet, and stress control. As with all other chapters, they will include many and varied case histories and ideas for what *you* can do to control and prevent endometriosis. I will offer information on the more conservative approaches and most recent developments in treating the disease with drugs and hormones. If you favor holistic methods of treatment, you will find what you require in terms of diet changes and alternate medical departures (such as acupuncture, herbal remedies, vitamin therapy, and relaxation techniques) that are equally effective in many cases.

Since endometriosis is responsible for up to 75 percent of all cases of infertility, I have prepared a special chapter on this widespread problem. Chapter 12 will take you on a comprehensive journey into the problems of infertility and what can be done for women so afflicted. Surgery is always a possibility with endometriosis and chapter 13 will divulge what happens when a woman surrenders to a doctor's advice for radical surgery to "cure" endometriosis. Women will tell their own stories—some of them happy that they had the surgery; some of them regretting it.

Since a large part of curing endometriosis depends on you, the last chapter will direct you to other women, lay organizations, and medically affiliated groups who keep up with the latest information on the problem. How important these groups are! For one, women who have experience in finding the right doctor can advise you on whom to see in your area. Women who may live in small communities can use these organizations to communicate with other women who share a similar medical history. Knowing that others are so generous with their support is as healing as any drug.

What the voices in this book tell about endometriosis is moving and compelling. I feel grateful to all the women who have helped me understand the disease. Their questions have inspired me to continue research into an early cure. I know it's possible. I just have to look at how far we've come in conquering this disease in the last decade alone. I feel certain we can win this battle together.

CHAPTER 3

The Hidden Disease: Why Doctors Fail to Discover Endometriosis

ON a warm day in April, two women working together at a television station decide to have a light lunch at a nearby sidewalk café. It's a friendly, crowded place, with small round tables set close to each other. Barbara, usually the more easygoing of the two women, seems worried as she leans forward and remarks to Jane: "Laura could lose her shot for a job in the newsroom. She's missed so much work lately. Maybe she doesn't want the job at all."

Jane: Between us, it's not the job. Laura's always in pain . . . she's got some real problems.

Barbara: What do you mean by problems?

Jane: She has endometriosis.

Barbara: What's *that?*

Jane: For years, Laura had terrible cramps and pain, but no doctor could tell her what was wrong. Now it seems that the disease has done so much internal damage that she can't get pregnant. *Endometriosis spreads!*

Barbara: How? Is it some new type of V.D.?

Jane: No, it's not a disease you can catch. That's all I know for sure.

A conversation like this one was exchanged over lunch somewhere in Manhattan, but one could easily find "Barbara" and "Jane" meeting at any coffee shop, discussing the plight of "Laura." Such conversations are no longer isolated cases, because the subject—endometriosis—has tragically become a widespread topic. Compassionate friends like Barbara and Jane can only begin to describe the extent of the disease's symptoms and effects. Every day in every city, millions of concerned women who know someone with endometriosis or who are themselves plagued by it are also searching for solutions to this new and growing health problem.

Who are these women?

One might be a friend, a boss, a relative—or she might be *you*. The facts now tell the story: a conservative estimate counts 20 million women with endometriosis, but realistically, there are more than twice that number of victims at varying stages of the disease. Millions of Lauras face the possibility of infertility and needless suffering. Millions more are crippled by relentless pelvic pain and its complications, such as debilitating cramps and bladder disorders. Some have lost faith in professional medical care, as one doctor after the other failed to diagnose their disease before it grew out of control. More important, vast numbers of women may have endometriosis and not know that they do.

THE TRAGEDY OF DELAYED DIAGNOSIS

It doesn't seem possible to have a progressive, chronic condition and not be aware of it, but with endometriosis this can happen. A sufferer may consult an unsympathetic doctor or a practitioner inexperienced in diagnosing or treating the disease. For her pain, she may be dismissed—told that her symptoms are all in her head or that they are blown out of proportion. The chief complaint—pelvic pain—is, however, not psychosomatic at all, but a *very real* characteristic sign of the disease.

Victims of endometriosis experience an unnatural biological phenomenon: the misplacement of endometrial cells that normally line the uterine cavity. These cells are pushed backward from the uterus during menstruation and run wild, implanting themselves on pelvic organs, where they not only grow but proliferate. Eventually, clumps of endometrial masses spread more and more with each menstrual cycle, contorting organs and making normal functioning difficult or impossible. This invasive process results in severe cramps, pain, and, if

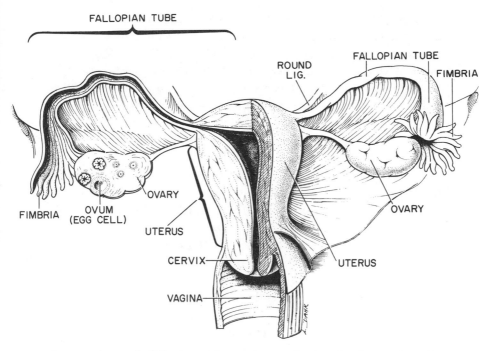

FALLOPIAN TUBE

ROUND LIG.

FALLOPIAN TUBE

FIMBRIA

OVARY

OVARY

FIMBRIA

OVUM (EGG CELL)

UTERUS

UTERUS

CERVIX

VAGINA

the ovaries and fallopian tubes are gravely involved, sterility. (See illustration, which shows the normal relationship of organs.)

Along the way, women who suffer from endometriosis often are subjected repeatedly to unnecessary surgery, endure years of drug therapy that may not be of much benefit or can even worsen the disorder, develop other stress-related problems from unrelenting abdominal discomfort, and relinquish chances for fulfilling personal and professional goals because of ill health.

Although I've never met Laura, I have a good sense of the misery she must be experiencing as a result of the ravaging effects of this disease. Not a week goes by that I don't see new patients who have come to me because they have been told by other doctors that the chronic pain from which they suffer is not real.

Dr. Donald Chatman, an obstetrician and gynecologist at the Michael Reese Hospital and Medical Center in Chicago, specializes in treating women with pelvic pain. He, too, is concerned that a problem exists in medical circles when it comes to understanding this disease. "There is no question that endometriosis is often misdiagnosed or underdiagnosed," he told me. "Primarily, I think physicians are not aware of the potential presence of the disease. For example, a mother calls her doctor and says, 'My teenage daughter has recurrent menstrual pain.' He might well say, 'That's a woman's curse,' and prescribe a drug like ibuprofen or Motrin and assume the girl's pain is of no consequence. Similarly, a woman in her thirties with severe menstrual pain can face the same kind of put-off response when she sees her gynecologist. I think doctors are not paying enough attention to the fact that a significant number of women are *disabled* by pain associated with the disease. A lot more research needs to be done to help them."

Misdiagnosis is predictable when physicians don't have the heightened awareness needed to make the correct diagnosis. In fact, a study was done on pelvic inflammatory disease (PID), a sexually transmitted disorder, in which it was found that the error rate of diagnosis was 35 to 50 percent! Many of those women actually had endometriosis, not PID.

My own extensive research and clinical experiences point up a second unfortunate complication: doctors may not address endometriosis in reference to debilitating pain as willingly as they will acknowledge the link between endometriosis and infertility. In effect, this is tantamount to denying that pain is as great a complication as not being able to conceive. I have discovered that women will suffer from wrenching pain for *years* before seeking treatment. Too frequently, it is the complications of infertility that bring them to their doctors. I have also treated young career women, full of dreams of their futures, who feel stricken, their energy depleted by months or years of having been incorrectly treated for "bladder infections" or "venereal disease," when their complaints, in truth, were caused by endometriosis. Victims of misdiagnosis write to me from all over the world—some of them women in their early twenties—describing in vivid detail the tragic and extreme "cure" a doctor has recommended: hysterectomy.

A Shocking Cure

A very distressing—and far too typical—letter came to me recently from a woman in Ohio, written on the eve of her twenty-sixth birthday. Karen described her tangled history with endometriosis, beginning with her final decision: the prior week, she wrote, she had signed a document giving her doctor the right to perform surgery to "clean up the endometriosis and save as much of my organs as possible." Her letter went on to detail her story:

For two years she had suffered from cramps, bleeding, and intense abdominal pain. One afternoon a cyst ruptured as she was driving to work. Miraculously, she got herself out of the car and flagged down a good Samaritan who took her to a hospital, where she was given emergency surgery.

At this point, Karen did not know she had endometriosis. After surgery, her doctor put her on tranquilizers for her continuing pain; then he followed up with hormone treatments to quell her menstrual cramps. She subsequently had two miscarriages and her doctor ran some tests on her, including a laparoscopy (the surgical procedure that enables doctors to see into the pelvic area). It was *then* finally that he discovered endometriosis!

"My doctor was very comforting," Karen said in her letter, "and I've always trusted him. He said there was a slim chance that I'd need a hysterectomy, but he'd try to save what he could. Of course, I heard the words I wanted to hear: he'd save me. I woke up from surgery and he told me the news. He hadn't saved anything and he'd given me a hysterectomy. That ended it for my ever having children and I wasn't yet twenty-six years old! I felt as if I'd been butchered, like a human sacrifice! But if he said I *needed* a hysterectomy, who should I believe? He also said that, in another month, I would have to go on estrogen supplements since he had removed both my ovaries, too. Was he wrong? What would you do?"

This woman's castration was presented to her *after the fact* as the only answer to her problem. Her surgery was needless. Had she seen a specialist in endometriosis, I feel certain that she could have had a chance at recovery. Trusting her doctor may have given her a measure of comfort, but this was not enough. As I see it, when her doctor operated, he did not have the expertise to understand that the internal bleeding was caused by endometrial masses. Doctors who do not have a trained eye can miss the condition in its earliest stages, even when it is literally at their fingertips. They may mistake it for something else—an infection or even cancer. This doctor's choice of treatment—a complete hysterectomy—harks back to what was common practice over a decade ago for such "far-gone" cases. That this physician subsequently prescribed hormones in the form of estrogen replacement so soon after surgery indicates another gap in his knowledge. You'll learn more about this form of compounding an error of judgment in later chapters.

Karen's story is just one of the thousands of such cases that have come to my attention by letter or when I have lectured on endometriosis throughout the country. Each one of the thousands of women who suffer from endometriosis to whom I have spoken and whom I have treated has contributed something valuable to my insight and given me greater knowledge and understanding of this condition.

What, then, is this hidden disease, and why is it one of this decade's most perplexing health problems?

WOMEN THEN AND NOW

Endometriosis is a complex disease, most often affecting women with complex lives. In the past ten years there has been a startling increase of reported cases among women who have postponed motherhood to pursue careers or simply to bring home needed additional income. Although this ailment is not restricted to women who put professional achievement first (endometriosis can strike teenagers as young as thirteen, women with children, even women who have had hysterectomies), cases are significantly on the rise among career women.

In simpler cultures where age-old, traditional women's roles are still abided by, women bear their first child at an earlier age. They then breast-feed their child, conceive a second child, and the cycle begins again. Over their life-spans, women who have borne children at a younger age, or who eventually have larger families, are found to be less frequent victims of endometriosis. Statistics from medical experts in underdeveloped areas tend to bear this out. Over the last twenty years, however, as personal achievement for women in developed countries has become more defined by professional gains than by creating and rearing a family, the incidence of endometriosis has increased.

A different vision of her place in the world is one way the contemporary woman is set apart from her more traditional counterpart. A second yet equally significant difference is the number of menstrual periods today's woman will experience. By bearing more children at an earlier age and by breast-feeding them between pregnancies, the traditional woman has about *ten to fifteen times fewer* menstrual periods than today's career woman. Such a woman, in other words, has about 55 periods during her lifetime as compared with a woman who does not bear a child and may thus menstruate *550 times* until menopause.

Although endometriosis is directly linked to menstruation, I would like to note that its cessation by pregnancy is not a cure for the disease, as less-informed medical specialists once believed it was. Endometriosis is very insidious and may, ironically, spare women who

would appear to be very likely candidates—childless career women—
while it cripples others with less characteristic profiles.

EXPOSING THE HIDDEN DISEASE

Endometriosis has been studied by scientists over the years, all of
them seeking an absolute answer to the question every sufferer of the
disease asks her doctor: Why me? One theory, proposed by a Dr.
Sampson in the 1920s, is still widely accepted by the medical community; it is discussed fully in the upcoming chapter. Sampson's
theory provides an explanation as to *how* the endometrial implants
find their way into the abdominal cavity, but not *why* the implants
stick to organs and grow.

This is the crucial question: *Why do implants "take" with some women
and not with others?* Such is the continuing mystery of endometriosis.

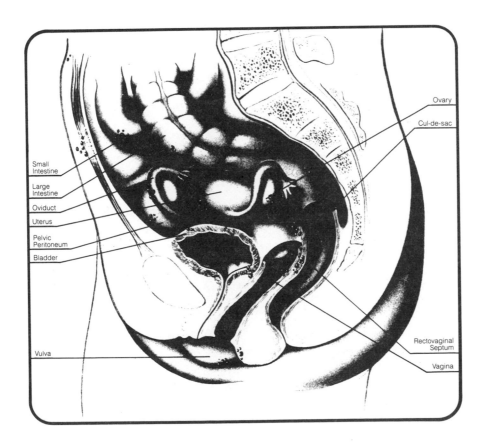

Four basic causes, which I will discuss in depth in chapter 5, have been pinpointed:

• *Hereditary factors.* You will be more likely to get endometriosis if close female relatives have had the condition, too. I personally would add to this a familial predisposition to menstrual cramps.

• *Immune system stress.* Endometrial implants may be more likely to proliferate when this infection-fighting system is weakened.

• *Hormone levels.* Higher estrogen and prostaglandin levels are associated with more cases of endometriosis and *pain* from the disease.

• *The embryonic theory.* One supposition is that you are born with the condition in a dormant state. If the internal environment is right, endometriosis will "take" and grow. (See illustration on page 21.)

No one knows precisely what combination of factors in what degree will create endometriosis, but I strongly believe that heredity and immune system stress are two major influences. One we cannot change, but the other—immune system stress—can be altered, and you will learn how to do this later on in this book.

We have come far in understanding this disease and the many almost miraculous ways to manage it. Before we talk about cures, though, let's take an in-depth look at the mechanics of endometriosis and its overall effect on a woman's body.

CHAPTER 4

Exposing the Hidden Disease

EVERY day in my medical practice I listen to women describe what it is that has brought them to my office. Sometimes the problem is clear to them—for example, they cannot conceive and fear they are infertile—though the *cause* has yet to be determined by me. Whatever the problem, I must probe for information that can direct me toward a cure.

In most cases I find that women have a fairly healthy sense of their own bodies; they are basically in touch with how they function. This is not as true, however, when the diagnosis is endometriosis. The response then is often confusion. Sufferers first wonder what this disease means, what changes have taken place in which organ and why, what they might have done to get the disease, and how they can be cured of it.

Endometriosis is directly connected to the uterus. But to fully understand endometriosis and how it claims its victims, we first have to understand menstruation—the cyclical process with which all women are familiar.

THE NORMAL MENSTRUAL CYCLE

During the second half of the menstrual cycle—the two weeks that begin with ovulation and end with menstruation—the endometrium, or lining of the uterus, prepares for conception. Activated by the ovarian hormones estrogen and progesterone, the lining becomes swollen with blood and glandular tissue. Estrogen, the first female hormone, essentially primes the body for ovulation and fertilization. Progesterone changes the uterine lining, preparing it for the eventuality of nourishing a fertilized egg by turning the lining soft and spongy and increasing it to about ten times its normal thickness.

The cycle begins this way: immediately after menstruation, the hormone FSH (follicle-stimulating hormone) is released from the pituitary gland and stimulates the ovaries to produce estrogen. On approximately the fourteenth day of the cycle, when the estrogen level is sufficiently high, a second hormone—LH, or luteinizing hormone—is released from the pituitary and triggers ovulation, that is, the release of the egg from the ovary. This egg is one of about four hundred eggs, from a reserve of almost half a million eggs, that will ripen during a woman's lifetime.

If the egg is not fertilized by sperm, resulting in pregnancy, the endometrium follows another course. First, the female sex hormones drop and a third hormone, prostaglandin, is released. Then the enriched endometrial tissue breaks down. The menstrual cycle starts as the uterus begins its rhythmic contractions. The unused endometrial tissue detaches from the womb and is normally flushed out of the body in the form of menstrual blood.

THE TRUTH ABOUT MENSTRUAL CRAMPS

In most women, uterine contractions simply press the sloughed-off endometrial tissue down its usual path through the mouth of the womb (the cervix) and out of the body via the vagina. The woman prone to endometriosis, however, experiences another phenomenon: because she may have a contracted uterus or a tight cervix, all the menstrual blood cannot easily flow out through the vagina. Rather, some of the blood-filled endometrium is forced up through the fallopian tubes, pushes backward out of the tubes, and is sprayed into the abdominal cavity, where it may attach itself to pelvic organs, producing the condition of endometriosis. Menstrual cramps and pain—

known technically as dysmenorrhea—the first symptoms of endometriosis, are the result of this retrograde menstrual bleeding.

Dr. John A. Sampson, a researcher and practitioner in Albany, New York, is responsible for naming the disease in 1927. Dr. Sampson theorized that this backing up of endometrial tissue, which he called retrograde menstruation, was the most probable cause of endometriosis. Dr. Sampson proposed an explanation as to *how* the endometrial tissue is flushed out of the fallopian tubes and into the abdominal cavity, but there is still no explanation for *why* the endometrial tissue implants itself in these abnormal sites.

It has been proved that nearly all women will experience retrograde menstruation, but that many women will reject the tissue while others become victims of endometriosis. Their implants "stick." Sampson's theory has yet to be disputed, although a number of other researchers have discovered immunological, hereditary, and structural connections, as well as a link between the amount of menstrual blood pushed through the tubes and the severity of the disease. I will investigate these factors in greater depth in the upcoming chapter.

The tragedy of this disease is that it can go undetected until it has done irreversible damage. Equally heartbreaking is a woman's fatalistic attitude toward menstrual cramps. When endometriosis takes hold, it has a distinct way of invading every aspect of a woman's life, and this invasion begins early on, with cramps. Most women who try to cope with monthly bouts of mild to severe and debilitating cramps will seek relief from the pain with familiar remedies: heating pads, hot water bottles, or over-the-counter painkillers like aspirin. They do not connect their cramps to any process *other* than menstruation.

It does not occur to them that they may have endometriosis because they do not know about it. Since they don't know how endometriosis can incapacitate their reproductive system as well as other organs, they don't seek medical help. But these women aren't to blame. More than likely, they have been taught that menstrual discomfort, like contractions during childbirth, is not only natural but part of being a woman. Where seeking medical help for childbirth is understood, consulting a doctor for "just cramps" is often considered frivolous and self-indulgent.

Complaints of pain from menstrual cramps were once considered a form of hysteria, not quite as counterfeit a condition as demonic possession, but close enough for disbelievers. The word *hysteria* is derived from the Greek word *hystero,* which means uterus. At one time, not long ago, it was common practice to ascribe metaphysical qualities to certain organs of the body, such as the heart representing love, the spleen connoting bad temper, and the uterus suggesting emotional problems.

Freud linked hysteria to sexual repression—a concept still revered by some medical doctors who mistakenly ascribe complaints of pain during a normal biological cycle to a woman's monthly compulsion to deny her femininity and her sexuality. In fact, women in *real* pain from menstrual cramps may be assailed by far more than a few days of infirmity a month. They may be suffering from endometriosis and their cries for help are being answered with outdated theories by physicians who do not understand the severity of their pain.

How do cramps occur and why do some women suffer from them over a lifetime while others never experience a single pang of monthly discomfort?

Physicians once pointed to a tight cervix as the probable and primary cause of menstrual cramps. They felt that this tightness obstructed the natural flow of blood out of the body. The treatment for a tight cervix—nearly totally out of use today—was a stretching procedure, a so-called dilation of the cervix. A series of surgical rods of increasing diameters were inserted into the uterus through the cervix. This stretching by larger and larger rods was thought to ease the suffering from severe cramps. Unfortunately, when the stretching procedure was halted, the cervix either healed back to its original size or, as a result of the scar tissue created by the treatment, became even tighter! Clearly, cervical stretching was not the answer for relieving or curing menstrual cramps.

Today we are aware that a tightened cervix may be less a structural problem than a chemical one. Cervical tightening as well as menstrual cramps has been traced definitely to hormone levels, most specifically to a third hormone group involved in menstruation: prostaglandins. There is now an undisputed correlation between menstrual cramping and the presence of high levels of prostaglandins in the female body.

PROSTAGLANDINS—THE NEW HORMONES

Prostaglandins, newly understood hormones, were first discovered and named in 1935 by Dr. U. S. von Euler, a distinguished professor and researcher at the Karolinska Institute in Stockholm. Dr. von Euler originally believed that these hormones were produced solely by the prostate gland in the male, which is his reason for naming them as he did. Continued research by a well-known group of Swedish scientists after World War II revealed more than fourteen different types of prostaglandins. Subsequently, in 1957, Dr. V. R. Pickles, a British physiologist at the University of Sheffield, conducted ground-breaking studies on the function and control of these amino acid–like hormones. Most significantly, Dr. Pickles found prostaglandins in uterine tissue. This discovery was a virtual medical milestone in the understanding of menstrual cramps.

About twenty different types of prostaglandins are found in nearly every cell and are responsible for many functions. As with any other hormone in the body, there are adverse side effects when prostaglandins are produced in overabundance. We are most concerned with the prostaglandin involved with menstruation, the one that causes uterine contractions: F2~ (or F2 Alpha). Normally, this hormone is kept in control by the "pregnancy" hormone, progesterone. If a woman conceives, she continues to secrete high levels of progesterone, and F2 Alpha is not released. The body supports conception by blocking prostaglandin production.

What happens if conception does not occur?

Prostaglandins released prior to and during menstruation stimulate *rhythmic contractions* of the uterus. These contractions help shed the uterine lining, causing menstruation. If the level of prostaglandins is higher than normal, menstruation will be accompanied by cruelly disabling cramps and other problems, such as headache, nausea, vomiting, diarrhea, lowered blood pressure, and even fainting spells and fever.

When Dr. Pickles and his team isolated prostaglandins—their so-called menstrual stimulant found in menstrual fluid—they were unable to provide a scientific answer to the question of why one woman secretes a higher level of this substance than another. We still have no satisfactory answer to that question. We can only suppose that, as with other types of body chemistry, such as having oily skin or a proclivity to slenderness, the answer lies in heredity. Whatever the "X" factor, it is proved that certain women will secrete more prostaglandins than others and that those women with *higher* prostaglandin levels will suffer from menstrual cramps *and* a tightening of the cervix.

When the cervix tightens, somewhat like a clenched fist, the flow of menstrual blood out of the body is obstructed. The blood, replete with prostaglandins, is trapped in the womb. The hormone is first absorbed by the uterine muscles, then released, *re*absorbed, and released again, creating a destructive and vicious cycle.

Unchecked, the prostaglandins circulate throughout the body without losing their potency. The uterus responds by contracting and cramping until the menstrual blood finally flows out from the vagina, carrying the prostaglandins with it. This release and absorption of prostaglandins can cause uterine contractions far more intense than labor pains during childbirth. There is also the likelihood that the menstrual blood that doesn't flow out of the body in a normal manner can back up into the fallopian tubes and then out into the abdominal cavity. This "backing up" eventually wreaks far greater havoc than excruciating menstrual cramps—it can lead to endometriosis.

Just as there is a correlation between high levels of prostaglandins and menstrual cramps, a similar relation exists between regularly painful menstrual cramps and the possibility of the onset of endometriosis. The issue is not, however, quite so simple. Severe cramps may be blatant signals of hormonal fluctuations, but they are not necessarily blatant warning signals to every woman—or physician—that endometriosis may be developing and spreading. In fact, many women who are spared monthly cramps go through life blissfully unaware that they are victims of endometriosis. For these women, endometriosis is finally diagnosed either when they complain of painful symptoms other than menstrual cramps or when they discover that they cannot conceive—or they miscarry. Let's take a closer look at this devastating illness.

DEMYSTIFYING ENDOMETRIOSIS

Endometriosis begins with a retrograde flushing of endometrial tissue that backs up into the fallopian tubes and then sprays into the abdominal cavity. The endometrial cells can then implant themselves on any organ—ovaries, fallopian tubes, bladder, bowel—and *grow* with each monthly cycle. One would guess that the endometrial tissue somehow gravitates toward its source, the uterus, and implants itself only there. This is not true. In a recent study by a team of endocrinologists and infertility specialists, led by Dr. Susan Jenkins at Duke University Medical Center in North Carolina, it was found that the ovaries were the most likely site of endometrial implants (nearly 60 percent of the cases). For unknown reasons, the left ovary was a more common site than the right by 20 percent. The uterus was the host organ in only 11 percent of the cases. The cul-de-sac, the cavity between the uterus and the rectum, also ranked high as a nesting location for these renegade cells. Endometriosis in the cul-de-sac can be responsible for lower back pain during menstruation. Cases are commonly found in which the bladder and kidney are involved. Still more surprising, but much more rare, has been the discovery of endometriosis in the lung, armpits, and brain. No women in this study were found to have implants on the cervix or in the vagina—in fact, implants in these two sites are nearly unknown.

Imagine now what happens every month when endometrial tissue, existing outside its normal environment, responds according to its nature. The vulnerable endometrial implants outside the uterus react to the surge of estrogen and progesterone. The tissue thickens and bleeds, as if it were growing in the uterus, but, unlike menstrual blood, it has no way to exit the body. The implants can enlarge and then cling to organs.

If the endometrial masses are not located near nerve endings, they may not cause pain. Endometriosis has been found in women who were pain-free and functioning normally, but who were suffering from other problems, such as uterine fibroids or infertility. About 30 percent of women with endometriosis have no overt symptoms and find out only incidentally that they have the disease. If the implants grow near nerve endings, however, a woman's life can be made miserable. Seventy percent of endometriosis victims may begin feeling pain about two weeks prior to and continuing into menstruation. Overwhelming damage can be done to organs bound with endometrial masses in both symptomatic and asymptomatic sufferers.

The most frequent complaint that leads me to suspect endometriosis in a patient is dysmenorrhea, or painful menstruation. Many women with endometriosis tell of long histories of menstrual distress, most specifically heavy menstrual flow accompanied by severe cramping. Backache and/or deep abdominal pain on either side of the body may indicate engorgement of blood in exiled endometrial tissue on the bowels or ovaries.

Dyspareunia, or painful intercourse, is yet another serious problem. Endometrial lesions, especially when they are trapped and growing in the cul-de-sac, can push the uterus into a retroverted position. Retroversion is a tilting back of the uterus. When the uterus is thus pulled out of its normal position, deep vaginal penetration during intercourse can be extremely painful.

Rectal bleeding, the need to urinate frequently, or blood in the urine during menstruation can also indicate endometriosis. Furthermore, if a woman feels pain radiating from her buttocks to the outside of her legs, her sciatic nerve may be affected. Vomiting and abdominal swelling may implicate the involvement of the small intestine. Finally,

SEVEN EARLY WARNING SYMPTOMS
OF ENDOMETRIOSIS

Many women are shocked by the diagnosis of endometriosis when they are tested for some other medical problem, such as recurrent bladder infections or an inability to become pregnant. A lack of symptoms (especially pain) may feel like a blessing. On the other hand, symptoms tell you that something is wrong, and you can wisely seek medical help before the disease grows out of control.

Studies indicate that most women with endometriosis suffer from two or more of the following telltale signs of the disease:

1. *Menstrual cramps that increase in severity over time.* Though progressively severe cramps are most common among women with endometriosis, cases also exist of patients who had serious menstrual cramps during their teenage years, then were spared for a decade or two until cramping returned when they were in their thirties.

2. *Intermenstrual pain, or mittelschmerz.* Midmonth ovulation usually causes no pain, but some women experience extreme discomfort at this time. Pelvic pain, lasting about two days, can be wrenching. Bleeding at the site of ovulation and subsequent irritation to intra-abdominal nerve endings are to blame. Mittelschmerz may be associated with light vaginal bleeding due to hormone changes and a midmonth shedding of uterine lining.

3. *Dyspareunia, or painful intercourse.* Recurring vaginal or pelvic pain during or after sexual intercourse may signal endometriosis.

4. *Infertility of unknown origin.* If you *have* been pregnant and cannot conceive now or, more likely, if you have never been pregnant and you are in your thirties or forties, you may have this disorder.

5. *"Bladder infections."* If you have been tested for urinary tract infections and all tests and cultures repeatedly come out negative, the problem might be endometriosis.

6. *Pelvic pain.* Do you notice pelvic pain that feels all-

encompassing a few days before and during your menstrual period? There may be incidents when intestines
seem involved, and other times when you feel definite
ovarian or uterine discomfort.

7. *History of ovarian cysts.* Doctors have found that
women with a tendency toward hemorrhagic cysts—ones
that tend to rupture and bleed—may also be more likely to
have endometriosis.

infertility, which may strike up to 75 percent of all women who have
endometriosis, is directly linked to this disease. Since the complications of endometriosis and its effect on fertility are so extensive, I have
devoted an entire upcoming chapter to describing this one aspect of
the disease.

Because endometriosis is so variable in nature, a small implant may
cause greater suffering than a larger mass. In either case, physical pain
from endometriosis does not exist in a vacuum. This physical pain
generally results in a life-changing state of emotional distress, a devastating side effect made worse by the belief among others—doctors,
family, friends—that the pain does not, in fact, exist.

Pelvic pain can become an overwhelming entity in itself. What
follows is the kind of story that describes, in part, what happens when
no one—boyfriends, emergency room doctors, gynecologists—believes a complaint of disabling pain. It's a story shared by many
women, and it was told to me by Alexa, a twenty-nine-year-old legal
secretary from Detroit.

Alexa's Story: "Endometriosis Destroyed My Chance for Marriage"

"To me, what's terrible is having the man you're about to marry
give up on you and walk out when you're sick and need him most.
What's worse is not being able to get a straight answer from *five*
doctors about why I was so sick. The combination of the two managed to leave me alone and in horrible pain for about a year. Finally, I
found out that endometriosis was the cause of it all.

"I never heard of this disease until a few months ago. It was
confirmed by the *sixth* doctor I went to and I wish I'd seen him before
Jack, my fiancé, took off. Jack was pretty fed up with me and my
condition and all our trips to emergency rooms, occasionally in the

middle of the night. I would double over with pain and sometimes could barely breathe.

"Jack said he loved me and that he'd do anything to help, but he didn't exactly love what he'd been hearing from the doctors: that my pain was from V.D.! It's humiliating to be told by three different doctors on three different occasions over eight months that your symptoms—most of all your *pain*—add up to an advanced stage of venereal disease. Especially when you're clean! Two other doctors treated me for a bladder disorder, vaginal infections, and once for a spastic colon. I had the feeling that they were wrong and that it was something deeper, more serious, but I didn't know why I felt that. It scared me.

"I was living on sulfa drugs, antibiotics, and assorted painkillers. The severest pain lasted about three or four days. Then I'd feel achy, and then okay for a while. I heard from a friend that orgasm relieved pelvic tension, so I'd try to be more sexually active. The irony was that intercourse hurt, leaving both Jack and me frustrated and angry. Jack was beginning to accuse me of faking the pain *and* cheating on him. It was the last test, the one for chlamydia, that did it for Jack. His sympathy had been strained to the limit and he left me. The pain increased in frequency and duration.

"About six months ago, I was telling a friend and her sister about the problem and I got an answer! My friend's sister was a sufferer, too. She'd been through *ten years* of misery and suffered the loss of an ovary, and she still had some problems. She said she felt as if she were reliving her own history by listening to me. When I heard about endometriosis for the first time, the pain made sense. I finally felt I had a chance."

It's always sad to hear such stories of women who don't get any emotional support or effective medical care for long periods of time. Not once was Alexa's pain taken seriously. This, to me, is the real crisis in diagnosing endometriosis. What is the problem?

PAIN AND EMOTIONAL TURMOIL

The human body was created with pain receptors. Without them we could not survive. Pain receptors tell us, for example, when to pull our hand from a dangerously hot object. Should we come into contact with something and it pierces our skin, pain receptors tell us we are bleeding and need first aid. Pain receptors also alert us when internal organs misfunction—heads ache, kidneys throb, throats burn, a uterus cramps. Everyone knows what most of such pain is like, but it can be difficult for a person who has never experienced a wrenching, disabling pain to comprehend another's misery. A knowledge of biology, a degree from a medical school, or even compassion for another human being cannot always guarantee either understanding or correct treatment.

Why is pain such a mystery?

An individual's response to bodily pain is always unique because pain is supremely subjective. Two people may be able to agree with each other about what a headache feels like and that childbirth usually causes more physical distress than a routine internal examination. They may not, however, agree about exactly which sensations and what degree of intensity constitute acute pain or an odd and persistent ache.

Each of us has a different pain threshold, which is a combination of psychological and neurological factors. At one extreme, stoics and mind-control practitioners may choose to feel no pain—some can even staunch the flow of blood from a wound by use of willpower alone. At the other extreme, hypochondriacs fervently believe in their suffering, and encourage it or create new illness. Most people fall somewhere between these two extremes. Whatever the pain—acute, throbbing, stabbing, burning, dull, aching—they can describe it accurately enough in all its varying degrees and severity so that others can understand.

This ability to communicate a private sense of pain to another gives us a chance to obtain medical help in a manner that is most effective. But what happens when communication is thwarted by a physician who *invalidates* a patient's report of pain, thereby invalidating the cause?

For women who have been told by doctors again and again that the pain they feel *does not exist,* emotional turmoil may become as much a symptom of endometriosis as the actual physical disability. As a palliative, unsympathetic doctors may prescribe Valium or other tranquilizers. Generally, when the pain persists, another doctor is consulted. Should he concur with the first, he may simply prescribe stronger tranquilizers, and a woman's illness becomes doubly wearing. Her self-doubt begins to grow as her pain increases in severity. The questions such a victim asks herself, however, remain unanswered: "How can I be creating such horrible pain? Since doctors tell me that I am to blame, how can I stop doing this to myself?"

Clearly, this situation is emotionally wrenching. Rather than follow their own inner voices, which know that this pain means something, these women are made to feel defeated, somehow responsible—and guilty—until the disease becomes so advanced and so serious that even a minimally experienced physician is finally able to diagnose it.

The Burden of Guilt

It is not only women whose endometriosis has been either undiagnosed or misdiagnosed who experience such self-recriminating attitudes. Even when endometriosis is properly diagnosed at an early stage, many women still wonder if there is a psychological cause of the disease and feel guilty that they have developed endometriosis. They often believe that they have "given" themselves endometriosis by subconsciously implanting these renegade cells. In either case, repeatedly having the *reality* of her pelvic pain denied leads a woman to develop a sense of self-blame.

Rona Silverton, a New York–based psychotherapist with analytic training, is documenting women's emotional reactions to endometriosis and what they can do to help themselves combat the problem. She sees in victims a common trait: self-blame and a sense of helplessness. Dr. Silverton notes: "If you don't have the reality of endometriosis confirmed, or if it's taking a long time to have it diagnosed, it stirs up other fantasies of what might be wrong.

"Some women fear they have a cancerous condition; others believe their pain is imaginary and don't seek further help. Some even think they're being punished for something they've done in the past. One woman—a professional now in her thirties diagnosed with endometriosis—confessed to me that she had had an abortion when she was younger. She believed her condition was related to her once having aborted a child. *Logically,* she knew hers was a physiological problem, but inwardly—for her—endometriosis was indisputably related to that abortion."

Personalizing the disease is only one of many reactions. One can almost understand how a sufferer could eventually declare a moral judgment on an illness, especially when she starts out being told the pain is imaginary. Since endometriosis does not present itself like a broken leg—that is, in an absolute and obvious manner—it allows for a wider margin of self-doubt if the doctor asserts that there is nothing wrong.

While coping with pain she doesn't understand, a woman's sense of doubt can be compounded by the fear of what can happen next.

There's a flood of feeling, especially about recovering and having children. Dr. Silverton reflected, "But there *is* hope, I feel. Once the disease is legitimized by virtue of correct diagnosis, and the reason she is in pain becomes clear, then [a woman] can take steps to relieve it. Counseling helps women sort out the physical symptoms and reduce some of the guilt involved."

To restore self-esteem, any woman with endometriosis must be educated about the disease, not only in terms of hard medical information but also with a conviction to heed her own inner perceptions. A woman may know she has endometriosis even though her doctor insists she does not! When this occurs, stories such as the following are common.

Betty's Story: Four Doctors, Five Different Diagnoses, Fifteen Months of Pain

Betty came to see me after she'd heard me lecture at a women's-interest group that focused on contemporary health issues. She told me her recent medical history, and I was shocked at how, in her case, doctors seemed to treat the *symptoms rather than the source* of pain. This is what happened as she tells it:

"I'm thirty-eight years old, and for most of my life, I've been healthy. When I got married thirteen years ago, my husband and I decided not to have children and I've never been pregnant. About fifteen months ago, life changed for me. One morning I awakened with a burning pain and a feeling of vaginal pressure. I went to my gynecologist, who diagnosed vaginitis. To be certain, he took a few cultures, which came up negative. I was still in pain, but he had no solutions for me, and in fact, things got worse.

"I went to another doctor. He was cold and unsympathetic, and he tested me for chlamydia, a venereal disease. That test came out negative, too. He seemed to be annoyed with me and prescribed a series of creams and vaginal suppositories, which were useless. I began feeling worse, this time with rectal pain.

"I found a third gynecologist and this one said I was suffering from a 'virus in the cells.' Don't ask me what this means because, with all his medical double-talk, I couldn't get a clear answer from him. This doctor played around with pills and oral medication for a 'fungus infection' that he next decided I had. I was in horrible pain—in addition to having menstrual cramps—and so he did a sonogram. It showed nothing.

35

"Five months had now passed and the pain began to shift, this time clearly to my urinary tract. I went to a urologist who said I had stenosis [a narrowing] of the urethra. He dilated my urethra, a procedure which was a nightmare and caused tremendous pain. He also gave me a cream, which didn't help. Worse, now—along with everything else—intercourse was painful!

"Confused, I actually went back to the second doctor I'd seen, who told me my uterus was *suddenly* tipping backward. He put me on Danocrine, which is a drug to suppress the disease, and after a few months on it, I'm beginning to feel better.

"In all, I saw four doctors. I felt they never took my pain seriously until a year had passed and a laparoscopy proved that something was actually there. I feel such frustration over this since I know I'd have been in much better shape if the first doctor had taken me seriously and had known about endometriosis."

TREATING THE SYMPTOMS, NOT THE SOURCE: ONE MEDICAL MISTAKE

What happened to Betty sometimes occurs when doctors focus on the most obvious sites of pain. We know that vaginal pain need not always indicate a localized infection, just as pain during urination need not only implicate the urinary tract. In Betty's case, four doctors held too narrow a vision of her many symptoms and long bouts of discomfort.

Betty was temporarily helped by the various drugs she was given, but it was not because the drugs cleared up the problem, as an antibiotic would destroy invading bacteria in the body. She was, in fact, *healing herself,* because the body is a perfect self-healing organism. It works like this:

In many cases, women with endometriosis reach a peak of pain and discomfort before menstruation. If the symptoms are misdiagnosed and treated as if they indicated another disease, such as a vaginal infection, a woman might indeed feel better after taking a drug. Why? As the menstrual cycle wanes and hormone levels equalize, there will usually be fewer pain-related symptoms. With or without the drugs, Betty would have felt better anyway! Her body actually was stabilizing itself naturally—or attempting to—until the next midcycle, when the hormones would again begin to rise. At that point, a woman in Betty's situation might be advised to take a drug such as Pyridium, which often is prescribed for bladder infections. Pyridium has the ability to numb the bladder and urethra; it also has the ability to mislead patients into believing they have been cured when they did not, in fact, need the drug in the first place!

Bladder infections can be tremendously devastating in terms of the pain in testing and the extensive financial and emotional costs of treatment. In truth, when Betty's test came back negative, her doctors should have thought of differential diagnosis—a system used to analyze a patient's problem. Combinations of symptoms may apply to one disease as easily as to another, but upon closer examination and questioning, there will be *other* critical symptoms that will clearly differentiate one disease from another.

Betty, then, was not suffering from infections in any pelvic organ, but from endometriosis, which her doctor discovered only upon performing surgery. In her way, Betty presented a characteristic profile of a potential victim of endometriosis: at the age of thirty-eight, she had never been pregnant; she was career-oriented, led a highly stressful life, and lately, she had suffered from bouts of menstrual cramps. Finally, she was given the drug Danocrine, which would give her pelvic rest and stop her menstrual fluctuations and, with that, her pain. (I will describe later the many hormone treatments for endometriosis, including Danocrine—a breakthrough drug in helping sufferers of this disease.)

When I saw Betty in her first consultation with me, I agreed that she needed treatment with Danocrine for at least six months. Along with this hormone treatment, I placed Betty on a diet devised to keep the body in a balanced state. Besides being nutritionally correct, the diet eliminated foods that have been specifically shown to increase or alter hormone levels. (Details about this regimen appear in chapters 9 and 10.) I examined her again after six months to see if the disease had been halted; there was a significant improvement, she no longer suffered debilitating pain, especially from menstrual cramps. At this point, Betty is on a low dosage of oral contraceptives—another treatment to be taken for about a year—and continuing with my diet.

TAKING CHARGE

Accurate information about the condition and an understanding of why doctors may be confused and fail to diagnose endometriosis will make a difference for any woman who suffers from the malady. Armed with knowledge, a woman with endometriosis can head toward a normal, joyous, and fulfilling life.

Right now we must think in terms of early detection. This is my goal, and it is a mighty one. Statistics are climbing daily as endometriosis appears to be reaching epidemic proportions. If you are a woman with endometriosis or believe you may have it, you *can* combat the disease and end needless suffering. Be informed (knowledge is power), be in touch with your body, *don't deny* symptoms but tend to them, and, finally, foster caring teamwork among your family, friends, and the physicians who treat endometriosis patients.

Women can become responsible partners with their doctors in obtaining the optimum health care they deserve. This book, I hope, will give you the tools you need to triumph over this disease.

CHAPTER 5

Who Gets Endometriosis and Why

HOW did I get endometriosis?" women want to know. "Why me?"

"Why is one woman susceptible to the disease and not another?" doctors ask.

Endometriosis is not a disease with a single cause. Clinicians have long been attempting to find the key to the onset of endometriosis. Is it associated with a virus, a weakness in the immune system, a hereditary predisposition, or is it related to personality—especially in regard to coping with stress or numerous other environmental variables?

Further probing brings up other questions of why one woman will fall victim to endometriosis and not another: Is the susceptibility traceable to a balance, or imbalance, of some combination of factors? Can you accidentally give yourself endometriosis as the result of a fall or any other accident? How implicated are birth control pills or even intrauterine influences from before you were born?

Ingenious laboratory experiments and dedicated scientific observations over the last decade have added to a vast body of knowledge about the disease. We have solved a few intriguing riddles about this condition, although we are still puzzling through the many possible theories. Of them, a number have been scientifically validated; others are myths—or misinformation—but they tend to hold a certain power for believers. In drawing together these many theories for you, I will tell you what doctors know at this point.

There could be no better time than now to find the cause and cure of endometriosis. Women understand their bodies and are more informed partners in their health care. This is an extraordinary time in women's lives. Contemporary pressures and biological nuances—such as high-pressure life-styles and the problems of delaying childbirth, in combination with abnormal menstrual bleeding—have significantly added to the number of victims of endometriosis. Overwork, worry, fatigue, and stress-related illnesses common to working women also contribute to the onset of the disease.

I treat sufferers of this disease every day. I can't help but feel admiration when women realize it is their right to ask questions and learn what they can to *fight back*. They want to know *why* they have what one medical journal called "the disease of the twentieth century." The answer, I am confident, lies somewhere in the etiology of endometriosis that follows.

ENDOMETRIOSIS: THE NEW DISEASE THAT'S OLDER THAN EVE

I feel certain that endometriosis affected regularly menstruating women before *Homo sapiens* discovered how to control fire or chip a block of stone into a working wheel. Though we have no way of knowing how earliest woman coped with menstrually related distress, we might guess that she believed the cause was cosmological and out of her control. The early Egyptians, who created one of the most advanced cultures four and five thousand years ago, were diligent recorders of history, astronomy, and science. It was they who for the first time made reference to a "painful disorder of her menstruation," duly noted on the Papyrus Ebers from the year 1600 B.C.

We are without further medical identification of the disorder until 1696, when the French surgeon Saviard noted the presence of endometrial tissue outside the uterus. Then in 1835 another French doctor, Jean Cruveilhier, described uterine cysts. Twenty-five years later, Dr. K. von Rokitansky, a German doctor, published the first paper on the disease, referring to it as an "adenomyoma," now called adenomyosis, or endometriosis confined entirely to the muscle wall of the uterus. At the turn of the century, two American doctors further described degrees of the disease, but it was not until 1921 that Dr. Sampson, as noted earlier, recorded his theory of how endometrial tissue implants on internal organs.

SAMPSON'S THEORY OF RETROGRADE MENSTRUATION

Sampson stated that menstrual blood containing viable fragments of endometrial tissue—the lining of the uterus—was "regurgitated" through the fallopian tubes into the abdominal cavity. Later laboratory experiments and observations of patients during abdominal surgery disclosed that most women have retrograde menstruation, but only a percentage will become victims of endometriosis.

Recent probes into the theory of retrograde menstruation reveal that a great percentage of women show an increased amount of blood in the pelvic cavity around menstruation and after ovulation. Blood has even been present in the dialysate (liquid drawn from the abdominal cavity) of women undergoing kidney dialysis while they had their periods. What this proves, again and again, is that retrograde menstruation is common.

Earlier experiments, specifically those performed in the 1950s, were more aggressive. One team—doctors R. B. Scott, R. W. TeLinde, and L. R. Wharton, Jr., of Chicago's Northwestern Medical Center— created pelvic endometriosis in rhesus monkeys by inducing retrograde menstruation in an extreme manner. Basically, what they did was cut into the monkey's uterus, opening it so that menstrual blood spilled directly into the pelvic cavity instead of being washed out through the vagina. Six of the ten experimental monkeys developed endometriosis—some within two and a half months, whereas others had no signs of it for nearly three years. In 1958 a number of women voluntarily submitted to an experiment wherein doctors injected endometrial cells into a laparotomy incision. This experiment also produced endometriosis in most women.

Sampson's theory has found a few detractors, but most doctors agree that the backward spraying of menstrual blood places endometrial tissue on vulnerable organs. Even Sampson postulated that in all probability there is "more than one" avenue available for the development and spread of this disease. One conclusion was that, he wrote, "the invasion and dissemination of endometrial tissue employ the same channels as the invasion of cancer." This meant that fragments of endometrial tissue reached other parts of the body through channels such as the blood and lymph systems. The actual process of tissue transference from one organ to another by blood or lymph glands is known as metastasis.

ENDOMETRIOSIS AND CANCER:
HOW THEY DIFFER

Sampson's theory brought up suggestions that other similarities existed between endometriosis and cancer besides the manner of transport of cells through the body. Yet both conditions differ significantly in manner and influence of growth, and in their effect on the host organs. The confusion begins, then, with the actual attributes of the two conditions.

When cancer cells find a host organ, the disease can consume the organ to which it has attached itself. Endometriosis on the other hand, is most often symbiotic. It exists on its own terms while using the host organ as a nesting place. Endometriotic cells will not devour host organs. Rather, endometriosis recalls the properties of a high-density glue: organs can literally become stuck together. "Kissing ovaries" is a picturesque description of an extreme case of endometriosis. The ovaries adhere to each other and also fix themselves to the posterior cul-de-sac.

Endometriosis apparently depends on the process of menstruation and implicates prostaglandin levels and ovarian function. Estrogen, viruses, and numerous other variable factors have been identified in the onset of cancers of the female reproductive tract.

The growth pattern of each disease contributes the third key difference between them. Endometriosis, in most cases, spreads rapidly, and will lead to a buildup of cysts or masses in the pelvis. Because it grows rapidly, it is often associated with extreme pain. The size of an endometriotic lesion does not determine *how much* pain a woman will feel; as we observed, microscopic endometrial implants on or near nerve endings can cause greater pain than much larger growths. In contrast, most uterine cancers, or cancers of the female reproductive tract, will grow slowly and therefore cause little or no pain. This is often why cancer is difficult to diagnose. Cancer, obviously, can be life-threatening, but endometriosis, on the other hand, is rarely fatal.

Sampson's theory and the laboratory experiments with rhesus monkeys introduced a second important hypothesis on the cause of endometriosis: its link with immune system function, or *dys*function. More specifically, scientists asked, how different are the immune systems of women with endometriosis as compared with those of women who are free of the disease?

ENDOMETRIOSIS AND THE IMMUNE SYSTEM CONNECTION

The immune system is the body's warrior force. Without its strength, vigilance, and quick response in battling "invading foreign bodies," each of us could lose our lives to the most minor infection or irritation. Invading bacteria, viruses, pollen, allergens, or any substance the body responds to as a threat are dealt with through this complex network. When disease gets a foothold, it is because of a weakness at some point in the immune system defense. It is to this system that scientists are looking for the answer to the development of endometriosis.

The immune system has an awesome task, employing a force of "agents" to keep it operating at its peak. These agents fight disease and *remember* the type of invading microorganism so they can prevent reinfection. The system's guard consists of interferon, complex fighter cells that attack bacteria and viruses by destroying their ability to reproduce in the human body. Interferon responds first in fighting infection, slowing down the potency of invaders so the body can summon other defenses. Laboratory studies reveal that only four hours after infection the body begins its charge with interferon.

The suppport system has varied responsibility, but it operates as a strategic team. Phagocytes engulf and consume invaders, or antigens, and can prevent disease from spreading. Antibodies recognize intruding bodies, clamp on to them, and destroy them. T cell lymphocytes, which are derived from the thymus gland, and B cell lymphocytes, derived from bone marrow, also work in tandem. T cells will control and regulate antibodies; B cells perform the important function of binding with antigens (the enemies) to render them harmless.

When bodily tissue is invaded, substances are released into the blood that marshal white blood cells of a different nature: neutrophils and macrophages. Neutrophils can consume about twenty-five invaders, and macrophages can "eat" four times that amount before expiring from the toxins they've ingested. Macrophages also clean up blood and keep it healthier by consuming diseased or ineffective red blood cells. (In terms of endometriosis, macrophage count, for example, has been found to be *double* the normal amount in the cul-de-sacs of women with the disease.) Memory cells function after disease is fought off, recognizing invaders and acting quickly to prevent reinfection.

Individual immune systems, like any army—no matter how sweeping—can suffer losses or serious setbacks in defense efforts through stress, alcohol consumption, smoking (cigarettes or marijuana), drugs (recreational or medicinal), and even diets that are high in fat, sugar, and, recent studies have found, dairy products. An extreme form of immune system devastation is AIDS (acquired immune deficiency syndrome). Traced to a virus that begins a chain of destruction among these infection-fighting cells, victims of AIDS don't die from AIDS itself, but from diseases the body's immune system is powerless to fight.

Doctors have long speculated that there may be an altered cellular immune response among women who develop endometriosis. This alteration, they propose, might explain why the implants adhere and grow. Among the many studies done in this field, investigators sought to explore an immune system deficiency that may occur along with another factor, for example, excessive menstrual flow or malfunction of the fallopian tubes. Answers to many of these studies were inconclusive. It was found that there might be an immune system breakdown *or* physiological problems in a victim of endometriosis, or an immune system deficiency *and* another factor. Therefore, conditions explaining the cause of the disease might exist as mutually exclusive factors or they might in fact be interconnected. In other words, there is, so far, no conclusive answer.

Cellular Immunity

Other studies examined lymphocyte activity among sufferers of endometriosis. In one such study, it was postulated that if an immune system misfunction were entirely the cause, women with endometriosis would show a higher incidence of infectious diseases and cancer. Increased illness, however, seems *not* to be a factor among the women who participated in this study. Newer experiments have focused on the effect of the cellular antigen CA-125, a cell that acts like a foreign substance in the body. How this antigen is produced by the body is unknown.

Two particular studies, one conducted by Dr. Donald Pittaway and colleagues at the Bowman Grey School of Medicine in Winston-Salem, North Carolina, and the other by Dr. Phillip Patton and colleagues at Minnesota's Mayo Clinic, have both turned up evidence to show that women with advanced endometriosis had elevated levels of CA-125, as did women who had acute pelvic inflammatory disease

(PID) and unexplained infertility. However, patients with less advanced stages of the disease, and women who did not have endometriosis, tended to have similar and lower CA-125 levels. Still, these investigators believe, this antigen bears further study because of marked elevated levels of it in women with endometriosis. They are also looking for a possible test for detecting endometriosis by analyzing CA-125 levels, and antigenic proteins like it, in blood samples.

STRESS AND ENDOMETRIOSIS

Psychologists and psychiatrists have been examining the effects of stress on the immune system, and it is here, I strongly believe, that we may find some of the answer to the origins of endometriosis. How do we cope with stress? Do we feel reasonably able to deal effectively with the world and maintain a positive sense of self, or do we feel helpless, as if no effort can make a difference? What if endometriosis is the outcome of *the immune system's collapse of effort?*

In a study measuring the correlation between the psychological symptoms of stress to natural killer cell activity, Dr. Steven E. Locke at Beth Israel Hospital in Boston reported in *Psychosomatic Medicine* that "symptoms such as anxiety and depression may negatively affect immunity." Those who were good at coping with life's vicissitudes tended to have "significantly higher natural killer cell activity" than those who felt a greater lack of control over the environment.

Transcendental meditation, hypnosis, biofeedback (wherein one literally learns to control the calming alpha waves produced by the brain), guided imaging, and other mind-control techniques have been studied extensively in laboratories and hospitals. Cancer patients have used many of these techniques to reduce pain and, in some cases, to fire immune system regeneration—in effect, curing themselves, or creating an environment where cure is more possible. Stress, as such, is not a fixed quantity: what is negatively stressful for one person may be of little consequence to another. For now, much of the data indicates that stress *can* contribute to the onset of disease.

Women with endometriosis tend to lead stressful lives—this fact cannot be denied. A persuasive enough argument has been made, in my estimation, for sufferers of this disease to consider making changes in their lives as a means of controlling the disease. The chapter on alternate treatments, following shortly, will offer a number of self-help plans to build resistance to disease.

THE EMBRYONIC THEORY

Could you be born with cells that have within them the possibility of growing into a full-blown case of endometriosis? In answering this question, researchers noted that many women do not have any classical symptoms of endometriosis while having the disease. Another dilemma involved women who had undergone abdominal surgery; there it was found that masses had developed that contained endometriosis*like* cells. That is, these patients appeared to have the disease, but in fact, they did not. How might this happen?

Noteworthy embryological studies uncovered some fascinating evidence. During intrauterine life, the fetal reproductive organs germinate from different types of cells. Vaginal tissue originates from a different set of genetic blueprints than uterine tissue, although both organs have the quality and capability of, for example, elasticity to accommodate childbearing. These embryonic studies went on to show that the tissue lining the ovaries, the endometrium, and the peritoneum—the smooth, transparent, and highly sensitive membrane that lines the pelvic and abdominal cavity—all originated from the *same* embryonic cell membrane.

It was then postulated that some of these cells could be transformed into endometrial cells or endometrial*like* cells through repeated irritation, such as pelvic infections, or by hormonal stimulation. In many cases, the physiological result is identical to having actual endometrial cells run wild and implant themselves: pain, cramps, and possible infertility. This mimicking of the disease posed some conclusions that interest scientists. The story that follows reveals why.

Endometriosis and Men

About a year ago, I received a letter from an Oklahoma woman who told an odd tale of pain and suffering due to endometriosis. To my surprise, Mrs. Petersen's account was not about her daughter, her sister, mother, aunt, or a friend. Rather, the unsuspecting victim of this insidious disease was her husband, George.

"How could a man develop endometriosis?" she asked. "How did nature go so wrong in George's case?" Since neither she nor her stricken husband could justify the problem rationally—men, after all, do not menstruate—Mrs. Petersen wondered if perhaps *she* might have been somehow responsible for his plight. Of course, she was not to blame, since endometriosis is *not transmitted sexually,* nor is it a contagious disease in any way. Endometriosis is a rarity in men, and how it occurs among them may enlighten us in treating women.

George Petersen's bout with endometriosis unfolded in this astonishing letter: He was only forty years old when the first symptoms appeared. George was in generally good health, except for frequent and severe headaches, brought on, they thought, by stress; he had also succumbed to chronic bladder problems. "Our doctor said George had an enlarged prostate," Mrs. Petersen wrote, "and he never really felt at his best for nearly two years. It seemed like a terribly long time for us. Finally, he was told he had cancer of the prostate. It scared us, but at least we knew what was going on, terrible as it was."

George was assured that the recovery rate was high, she said, especially if the cancer was caught early. He agreed to the treatments that were advised, including a form of estrogen, which was supposed to shrink the tumor. About a year after George discontinued estrogen treatments, sharp abdominal pains began to plague him. George feared the cancer had returned, or worse, that perhaps it had spread from his prostate to other organs. He avoided medical care for a few months, until he collapsed one night in extreme pain.

"He managed to use the bathroom and urinated blood," Mrs. Petersen wrote. "This was a mournful night for us, since we feared the worst. I got George to a hospital and his doctor operated on him the following day." In surgery the doctor saw that the cancer was under control, but that there were many spots of endometriosis around his bladder! This is what caused him such crippling pain, along with other irritating symptoms.

George was probably born with dormant cells that, under the right conditions, developed and behaved *as if they were endometrial tissue.* He experienced the identical symptoms that women have with the disease. We know that estrogen is a factor in the growth of endometriotic tissue in women. If George stays off estrogen treatments, the endometriotic cells should shrink and the disease not recur.

To many scientists, this man's unique reaction and sensitivity to the hormone validates the embryonic theory of why endometriosis could develop in some individuals but not in others.

THE HEREDITY FACTOR: IS ENDOMETRIOSIS A FAMILY TRAIT?

"What are the chances of my passing this disease on to a daughter?" a patient asks me. At thirty-eight years old, Terri is pregnant for the first time after successfully battling endometriosis. A routine test—amniocentesis—has indicated she is carrying a girl. Terri fears that her child will suffer from the disease as she had.

Three weeks after I have diagnosed her case, a second patient says: "How did I get endometriosis? No one in my family has it but me." Joan fervently wants to know why she has been "singled out" by this disease, since her sisters and mother are free of it.

A third woman explains: "My mother was tortured by menstrual cramps and endometriosis until menopause. Through some miracle, I'm okay. She said I still could get it, too, that the real 'curse' is inheriting this kind of pain. Is my mother right?" Diana has been fortunate thus far, but she feels it's just a matter of time before the first symptom of the disease becomes apparent.

Nearly all my patients with endometriosis routinely ask questions like these; in fact, such questions are fundamental and make good sense. Could there be a strong hereditary component in a family's gene pool that determines which of its women will or will not develop endometriosis? Pursuing a genetic link to this disease may provide one kind of clue to its cause, and that pursuit begins with the most basic question: Why me?

In continuing efforts to track down the cause of endometriosis, modern scientists have tended to concentrate on the physiology and chemistry of the disease. They have only just begun to examine the role of heredity more intensively. Specifically, they are looking for evidence of tendencies toward the disease among female relatives on both the maternal and paternal sides of a family. So far, the key to determining whether a woman will develop the disease lies in her *inherited predisposition.*

Not all genes establish absolutes, such as curly hair, brown eyes, or the shape of fingernails. Some genes set a range of possibility or susceptibility, not an absolute number or condition. You may be genetically predisposed to weight gain, but your actual weight can be environmentally determined by caloric intake, general health, and a combination of personal and regional attitudes about being overweight. A similar type of range applies to predispositions to diseases such as diabetes, cancer, and endometriosis; important genetic clues have recently been found to common mental disorders, too, including Alzheimer's disease and manic-depressive illness.

Geneticists expect a simple test to be available in the future that will predict above average susceptibility to illnesses, both fatal and disabling, which no doubt could include genetic testing for endometriosis.

Imagine this: by the time such a genetic marker is found, not only could there be a cure for sufferers, but a preventive treatment might be available for those who *would* contract it! For now, a conjunction of heredity and environmental factors for millions of women has resulted in endometriosis—but each woman, I believe, still has some control over the management and cure of the disease, despite her family history.

The Incidence of Endometriosis Among Relatives

Who, then, is most likely to be a genetic candidate for the disease? Ten to twenty years ago (perhaps longer), the implicit assumption was that endometriosis was a disease carried by and exclusive to white middle-class women who were under stress and career-oriented. No real data was collected on the incidence of the disease within these women's families. Researchers simply tended to associate it with women who fit this characteristic scenario, and did not probe any further. The first real study was done privately in 1970 by Dr. Brooks Ranney, a South Dakota gynecologist, who first noticed a distinct biological pattern among his patients with endometriosis—many were related to each other. Dr. Ranney sent questionnaires to these women. Based on their responses, he calculated that 22 percent reported relatives (both near and distant) who had undergone surgery for endometriosis.

How coincidental is endometriosis among female relatives, and were Ranney's figures high or low for the general population? A study at Baylor College of Medicine, in Texas, in which 123 women participated, attempted to provide more conclusive evidence. In this 1980 study, researchers attempted to trace lineage patterns of the disease by classifying female relatives into categories, then looking at their medical histories. "First-degree" relatives were defined as mothers, daughters, and sisters; "second-degree" relatives included maternal grandmothers, aunts, and nieces; and "third-degree" relatives were female first cousins.

The results were telling: overall, the Baylor team estimated that women whose first-degree relatives developed endometriosis are *seven times more likely* to develop the disease. Of that percentage, *severe* endometriosis involved 61.1 percent of family-related cases and 23.8 percent of nonfamilial cases. This meant, clearly, that a woman whose mother or sister had severe endometriosis was a high-risk candidate for the disease and should be tested for early detection and treatment.

In 1986 another study, this one at the Medical College of Wisconsin, expanded on Baylor's investigation. This team added some interesting points. Of women participating in the study who reported other family members with endometriosis, about 79 percent of the cases involved maternal lineage and 7 percent implicated the father's side. Of the women studied, nearly 35 percent of mothers and 21 percent of sisters suffered from endometriosis, too. For second-degree relatives, numbers were significantly lower: for grandmothers the numbers were 0.4 percent, and for aunts the percentage tallied at 3.1 percent. (Such low numbers among an older generation do not necessarily mean lower incidence of the disease. This generation observed different conventions: they married younger and bore children at an earlier age. Fewer reported cases may have also had to do with fewer available diagnostic methods decades ago.)

What do these studies tell us about coincidence of the disease in families? *A hereditary factor does, obviously, exist, but it is not an exclusive indicator* of endometriosis. I suspect that there is a stronger hereditary predisposition toward menstrual cramps than endometriosis and that endometriosis may evolve with them. Heredity may be just part of the story, but I believe that there is a persuasive argument for making family histories an essential part of the diagnostic process.

THE HEREDITARY FACTOR II: ARE THERE RACIAL IMPLICATIONS?

We have to refer to the original supposition that only white middle-class women contract endometriosis to understand why some doctors have misunderstood racial distribution of this disease. Medical textbooks told them so. References to endometriosis tended to profile the "typical" patient, and, in nearly every case, she was the slightly privileged *white* woman. Endometriosis, then, had its own built-in bias, and in the minds of some doctors, it was as much a part of the diagnosis as any other telling symptom. This commitment to an outdated medical bias excluded black, Asian, Middle Eastern, and even Jewish women, among other ethnic groups. Doctors who treated such women dismissed the diagnosis of endometriosis—no matter how obvious a case it was—and assigned the condition another name. What were the fates of these patients?

Kayla fits this indicator perfectly. A former dancer, Kayla is a native Californian of Japanese and Korean extraction, now teaching in New

York and a patient of mine. She performed for ten years with a touring dance company, and many times she went on stage suffering from extreme pelvic pain. "The doctor said I had pelvic inflammatory disease, and that I'd probably gotten it from sexual contact with my boyfriend," she told me. "I took antibiotics again and again, but they helped only for a short time. When I quit the troupe to start teaching, I tried a different doctor. She said I had endometriosis, and she put me on hormone pills."

Being told that she had endometriosis was an unexpected revelation for Kayla. For nearly fifteen years, she was automatically diagnosed as having a sexually transmitted disease, and she believed it as fervently as she believed in the legitimacy of the medical system. Now she is questioning the diagnosis of endometriosis, even though she can measure the improvement in her health. What has happened is that Kayla's sense of self-esteem has suffered because her friends have told her that Asian women do not get endometriosis! She wants to know for certain what is wrong with her.

Kayla's dilemma has been common among other Asian women and more so among black women, many of whom have faced stereotyping in medical care. Kayla has endometriosis, not pelvic inflammatory disease. The difference between the two needs to be clarified. In endometriosis, pelvic organs can *appear* inflamed due to a reaction to the prostaglandins released by endometrial tissue. Endometriosis is *not* caused by or related to bacterial or viral infection; therefore, antibiotics will not help. Pelvic inflammatory disease (PID), in contrast, *is* caused by bacterial infection, which *will* inflame pelvic organs. If antibiotics are not given to control the disease, it can lead to progressively severe symptoms of pain and progressive damage to pelvic organs.

I cannot vouch for all other cases, but I venture to say that a large proportion of nonwhite women, like Kayla, have been misdiagnosed. Many doctors now, such as Dr. Donald Chatman in Chicago, are involved in intensive research that disproves prejudicial profiles of patients with the disease. Dr. Chatman has concentrated on the incidence of endometriosis among black women, who are most frequently misdiagnosed. Researchers in Israel, Japan, and China are also reevaluating data as cases of the disease increase in those countries.

Doctors in certain areas of this country do not see many cases of endometriosis and they may be confused when confronted with such patients, be they white, black, or Asian. Others, referring to an older text for guidance, accept the racial stereotype. But with an enigmatic disease like endometriosis, exceptions and modifying factors cross all racial lines.

If you are a black or Asian who tends toward menstrual cramps, often with increasing severity over time, if you are active sexually and experience pain during intercourse, and if you are of childbearing age and have never conceived—either with forethought or accidentally— you may have endometriosis. If doctors insist you are suffering from *recurring* viral infections of the bladder, pelvic inflammatory disease, or psychosomatic illness, do not hesitate to get a second or third opinion. Seek out doctors who are specialists in treating patients with this disease. Endometriosis doesn't discriminate!

CAN AN ABORTION TRIGGER ENDOMETRIOSIS?

Abortion is a delicate situation for even the most sophisticated of women. A universe of conscious and unconscious thoughts and feelings are connected with it. There often is an accompanying sense of fear (associated with the medical procedure itself) and a measure of sadness or guilt (linked to one's personal view of abortion). Although everyone differs in response, I have found that any woman who has had an abortion wonders how her health might be affected by the procedure: Will she be infection-free? Will abortion influence her ability to have children? Could it bring on some other as-yet-unnamed disease sometime in the future?

More to the point, women ask me, "Would I have endometriosis if I hadn't had an abortion?"

In evaluating my own work on the subject as well as the research of others, my scientific conclusion is this: endometriosis—as a consequence of abortion—is not an absolute biological inevitability. In fact, cases of abortion causing the disease are rare. When they do occur, it could directly involve an abortion technique, now out of favor, called hysterotomy.

Perhaps the best way to understand hysterotomy is to think of it as a mini-cesarean section. In this type of abortion, a small incision is made in the abdomen; then an internal incision is made in the womb and its contents are removed. Surgeons make a transverse (horizontal) or classical (vertical) incision in the lower portion or lower flap of the uterus—the same choice of incisions used for full-term deliveries by cesarean section. It is this type of surgical procedure, made during the late first trimester or early second trimester of pregnancy, that could be most responsible for the onset of endometriosis.

Why is this so? In the early months of pregnancy, there are still living endometriotic cells lining the uterus that have the potential to implant themselves on abdominal organs, and on the scar, given the chance. We know that pregnancy halts menstruation, which is the usual time of transport of these cells from the uterus. Therefore, another avenue into the abdominal cavity is required before any invasive endometriotic cells can run wild. Hysterotomy supplies the route. (Full-term cesarean deliveries differ entirely. At term, the placenta is fully formed and no endometriotic tissue remains in the uterus. Therefore, there is no way for random tissue to implant itself, or spread to an abdominal incision and implant itself there.)

Immediately following hysterotomy, surgeons will routinely cleanse the *internal* abdominal area of cells and blood clots with saline solution. However, in some cases, the cleansing is not effective enough; random cells that have been sprayed outward when the incision was made find a host organ. If the patient has a tendency toward endometriosis, the disease could take hold. (It is also possible that she already had endometriosis before the abortion, and the operation released other live cells.)

I had the occasion to treat a woman suffering from abortion-related endometriosis just recently. As much as I thought Mariska's story vivid and unique, she could be any other woman vulnerable to this disease.

Mariska came to see me soon after discovering a lump in a small abdominal scar above her pubic bone. The lump wasn't causing her any pain, she said, although she'd been feeling uncharacteristically tired early in the day, and her menstrual cramps were getting worse. When I took her medical history, I was surprised to hear that she had defected from Czechoslovakia with a friend five years before. She had been living in America for most of the time since defecting.

Mariska, I learned further, had been an idealistic nineteen-year-old Olympic ski-team hopeful when she was soundly blamed for "getting herself pregnant," then telling no one until she was three months along. The facts were a lot kinder than the wrath of her parents, her coach, and the team doctor, for she had no idea that she was going to have a baby.

Mariska, a strong downhill skier, had been training intensively since she was twelve years old. "I was physically at my peak of strength and flexibility," she said, "and I was told not to worry if my periods came irregularly." This is a common occurrence among many women in dance and sports. One side effect of the committed athlete is lowered estrogen levels, which can stop menstruation or significantly lighten menstrual flow. For Mariska, these hormonal changes were brought on by a low-fat diet, supplemented with a plentiful dosage of what she was told were "muscle-enhancing amino acids," along with a strenuous daily exercise regime. That she missed four consecutive periods therefore didn't alarm her, even though she had been having a sexual relationship for the first time. What she did find worrisome was the sudden bloating. That prompted her visit to the team doctor, who told her his findings.

Although she was against abortion for herself, Mariska was told to terminate the pregnancy. If she chose to keep the baby, all her training would be in vain—pregnant downhill skiers do not compete—and she'd upset team morale. Believing in the "infallibility of those who cared for me," Mariska agreed to a hysterotomy. Following surgery, she recovered quickly and competed in the Olympic Games.

I examined her six years after these events. I strongly suspected endometriosis, and this was doubly confirmed by laparoscopy. The disease had sprayed from the point of incision on her uterus to the scar on her abdomen. The endometriosis had also wrapped itself thickly around the fallopian tubes—not a good indicator for any woman who still wants children. I recommended treatment with Danocrine for six months and did exploratory surgery to remove as much endometriosis as was visible. It remains to be seen whether Mariska will be able to conceive.

Abortion by hysterotomy is rare now; doctors prefer other techniques that do not require uterine surgery.

CAN ENDOMETRIOSIS SPREAD DURING SURGERY?

In her letter to me, a twenty-eight-year-old Grand Rapids high school teacher wrote of her fears about undergoing surgery. It seems that Marilyn's reservations about having surgery—even though it was for diagnostic purposes only—were based on a misinformed connection to cancer. She wrote:

"My doctor feels I have endometriosis, but he wants to do surgery to confirm it. I'm worried that if I have surgery, the disease will only get worse. I have heard that endometriosis acts just like cancer. If you cut into it, the disease can spread because (1) some cells can get free from the tumor and infect other organs and (2) the cells are stimulated to grow from the oxygen in the air. Is there a way to confirm my endometriosis without the risk of making it worse?"

Marilyn's questions touch on two important issues involved in understanding and treating endometriosis. The first is the reason for surgical diagnosis, and the second involves the confusion between the pathology of cancer as one type of disease and endometriosis as another.

A woman's medical history in combination with her doctor's clinical findings might clearly indicate endometriosis, thereby making surgical diagnosis unnecessary. But this cannot always be the case. If a doctor is unsure of the diagnosis (especially when endometriosis is at an early stage of growth and does not yet produce large masses), or if he is unable to determine the nature of the tumor he feels while giving his patient an internal examination, he will want to do a laparoscopy. Although this is minor surgery (it will be discussed and illustrated in the next chapter), it is, for Marilyn and women like her, still an operation wherein something might go amiss.

There has been some documentation of endometriosis spreading as a result of laparoscopy, but this is rare and is most likely to occur when there is a history of *repeated* laparoscopies. In these cases, the endometriosis grows internally around the area of incision and implants itself in the scar, and a second or third incision in the same scar could free some cells. In a few cases, women who underwent surgery for hernias were later found to have endometriosis in the scar tissue.

If Marilyn's doctor feels that laparoscopy is called for, and there is no emergency, he might prescribe the medication Danocrine. This medication, as you will learn in a later chapter, renders endometriotic cells inactive. Taking Danocrine for a two-month period preceding laparoscopy should be sufficient to halt the growth of Marilyn's endometriosis, as well as lay to rest her fears about contamination during the procedure.

Cancer and endometriosis do not have much in common, other than their methods of invasion in the body. Cells of either type may use similar channels to reach internal organs such as the lymph system or the blood, or, after implanting themselves, cells may metastasize, or grow into a cyst or tumor. Endometrial cancer and endometriosis are not the same disease, although it has been found that childless women tend to be vulnerable to both conditions and that a great percentage of women with endometrial cancer suffer from menstrual irregularities.

My thought is that Marilyn might have seen endometriosis described as "benign cancer" and attached to it some faulty ideas about its growth patterns, such as by oxygenation. Endometriosis does not respond to temporary aeration because of an incision in the abdomen.

THE TAMPON DEBATE:
IS THERE A CONNECTION TO ENDOMETRIOSIS?

In my practice, numbers of women who use tampons exclusively (or use them in combination with pads for heavy flow) worry that tampons may be implicated in the onset and progressive growth of endometriosis. There are a number of reasons for their concern:

If tampons block menstrual flow and keep blood in the vagina, they ask, won't the tampon help push some of the blood back into the uterus?

What about the chance for infection? Aren't tampons actually an unsanitary way to manage menstrual flow? They remember the scare years ago from toxic shock syndrome and its connection to tampons.

Finally, they might add, "I know something is wrong because sometimes my body seems to expel a portion of the tampon naturally. Isn't this an indication that I might be doing something harmful to my health? Aren't pads the safer choice?"

These issues have all been scrutinized by gynecologists and clinicians studying every subtlety involved in endometriosis. One such study, conducted by Karen Lamb, Ph.D., and Nancy Berg at the Medical College of Wisconsin, investigated the tampon–endometriosis connection with nearly five hundred respondents who were members of the Endometriosis Association and sufferers of the disease. The study resulted in a number of conclusions. Among the most significant of them are these: tampon usage for women with endometriosis was not greater than rates for the general population, and, as yet, there is no clue to the role tampons play, if any, in the disease.

The cardboard-encased tampon was invented in 1933 by an ingenious Colorado physician. Tampax Incorporated, which bought the patent three years later, popularized the product almost single-handedly over the next thirty years or so. Other companies then entered the tampon market, introducing their own version of the original. Although today sanitary napkins outsell tampons by a small margin, to some women, tampons have the benefits of contained blood flow, comfort, and invisibility.

The tampon as we know it has not come this far without its own brand of controversy. The subject of some moral and scientific debate until the mid-1960s, the tampon triumphantly held its position as a safe and reliable women's hygiene product. Then in 1980 a sudden wave of toxic shock syndrome (TSS) mistakenly focused on tampons as the cause of this illness. One fact used for validation was that the illness seemed to strike white women, many of whom were menstruating at the time, and most of whom were using tampons. The Centers for Disease Control, though, noted that TSS also struck children, adolescents, and men and that the fatal cases crossed all age and sex lines. Eventually, clinicians postulated that immune systems in menstruating women are more vulnerable, which might account for the higher incidence among such victims.

Researchers into toxic shock syndrome, however, postulate one link between menstruation, tampons, and the illness. "Superabsorbent" tampons, most notably, expand to creat a pluglike effect, thereby trapping excess menstrual blood in a pool in the vagina. This pool of blood in combination with the blood-soaked tampon may in some cases create an airtight culture medium. In such an environment, bacteria might flourish and the toxin may develop. Another variable was found by researchers: tampons left in the vagina for periods of time greater than the four or five hours recommended (for example, those worn overnight) might cause abrasions, irritations, or sores in the vagina, thereby encouraging bacterial growth.

It is *because* tampons can stop the flow of menstrual blood out of the body that endometriosis sufferers bring up their first worry: couldn't a tampon somehow create enough mechanical pressure to flush blood back into the uterus? The answer is no! Once menstrual blood has passed through the cervix and enters the vagina, it will only leave the body. Since a tampon is placed in the lower part of the vagina, it does not block the blood's exit from the cervix. Although endometrial cells are sprayed into the abdomen by retrograde menstruation, tampons have no effect on the uterine contractions that propel the cells.

What of the feeling that the body expels tampons because they are unnatural devices? If endometriosis sufferers find that a tampon dislodges itself and moves down the vagina, the reason is tied to uterine contractions and menstrual cramps, not to "intuitive" biological knowledge. Women with endometriosis almost always have menstrual cramps, and these cramps exist in differing degrees of intensity. In fact, uterine contractions can even be measured on a scale. For example, the average force required to drive a baby out through the cervix is 50 millimeter mercury. The low end of the scale is 10 millimeter mercury. The force of severe menstrual cramps has been measured at 100 millimeter mercury. This gives you a good sense not only of the pain a woman will feel but of why a tampon would move down the vagina.

The wisest use of tampons is to change them every four or five hours, which gives the vagina a chance to cleanse itself, and to wear sanitary napkins overnight. Until further research is completed, 100 percent cotton tampons should be used, instead of those with synthetic fibers or deodorants.

COULD A SPORTING ACCIDENT CAUSE ENDOMETRIOSIS?

An interesting letter arrived from a woman in Colorado, posing a question that had not been asked of me in a long time. In her letter, Sherry said that she wanted to settle the nagging suspicion that endometriosis may have been induced through fate's intervention. She specifically referred to two accidents in her past, in which she had been struck forcefully in the abdomen.

"Maybe I'm grasping at straws," she wrote, "but I can't help wondering how I got endometriosis. There's nothing like it in my family and I seem to be the only woman I know of out here with the condition. Isn't there some likelihood that a shock to the system can start some internal chain reaction that brings on this disease?"

Sherry had been an active teenager, although menstrual cramps slowed her down through her high school years. During the last half of her senior year, her cramps worsened. Yet she suffered silently. "I was raised to be tough about things that made us physically and emotionally uncomfortable," she wrote. "It isn't unusual out here. This is a ranching community and life can be hard. No one cares about complainers." It was during a difficult bout with menstrual cramps that she played in a school volleyball competition and was struck by the ball as she jumped to hit it.

"I doubled over so suddenly, and I was in so much pain," she wrote, "that I had to be carried off the court. For days after that, I felt like I had to urinate all the time. The pain soon stopped, but my cramps started to get worse from about that time." Over-the-counter painkillers offered some relief while she waited to "grow out of" the problem. But it was not to be. Five years later, Sherry went on to say in her letter, she was horseback riding with her new husband when she was thrown by the horse, landing belly-down on a rock. This time, she began bleeding. Frightened, she went to a gynecologist.

Sherry was hospitalized and went into surgery for removal of an ovarian "chocolate cyst," a cyst with blood in it that has become dark brown and thick as tar. When a biopsy of the cyst was performed, it revealed endometriosis. Curious, Sherry asked her doctor if the first accident might have set off some "internal disorder" that fostered growth of the disease. It was the doctor's opinion that accidental traumas have no effect on the onset of endometriosis.

I have found no reference in any scientific journal that implicates any sort of trauma—such as being hit by a ball, falling off a horse, or being injured in an automobile accident—in the onset of endometriosis. In Sherry's case, the second accident only helped *identify* the disease. The fall ruptured an endometriotic cyst, which, upon rupturing, leaked blood over the pelvic organs, causing extreme pain. I would venture to say that since she suffered from menstrual cramps, the disease had most probably developed years before the incident on the volleyball court. The force of a ball or the hardness of a rock impacting on the abdomen might irritate the fine nerve tissue lining the peritoneum, but such an impact does not trigger the disease.

CAN BIRTH CONTROL PILLS CAUSE ENDOMETRIOSIS?

Jacqui is a patient who for years suffered from infertility problems related to endometriosis. After surgery and medication, she was able to conceive two children. Now it appears that her disease is under control. When Jacqui came for a routine examination last spring, she mentioned that her sister was taking high-dosage birth control pills.

"Franny has been telling me how bad she's been feeling," Jacqui said. "I think of myself when I hear her—I could swear that the symptoms sound just like she's got endometriosis. Franny never had any problems like cramps and pain before starting the Pill. She's got a bit of a weight problem, and that worries me, too. What are the chances that the Pill is giving her endometriosis?"

Birth control pills *do not cause* endometriosis. In fact, they were once considered the treatment of choice to control the disease. Oral contraceptives are a balance of estrogen and progesterone, and the pills vary in formula and dosage. Although we know that estrogen influences the *growth* of endometrial cells, it has not yet been implicated in creating mutant cells that may become endometriosis. Let's take the next step. If we examined under a microscope the endometrial tissue of women on oral contraceptives, we would find that the cells have become somewhat abnormal. This abnormality renders them inactive; that is, as a result of retrograde menstruation, they will not implant themselves on host organs and grow there.

In evaluating Franny's condition, I'd have to consider her weight problem along with her sister Jacqui's history of endometriosis. Overweight women are often more susceptible to diseases affecting the uterus. About half of all such women, in fact, have suffered from some form of uterine cancer. High-fat or cholesterol-laden foods are most responsible for weight gain, and researchers are finding that these treacherous fats have the ability to convert into estrogen or stimulate hormone production. Greater production of estrogen influences buildup of the endometrium, causing a heavier menstrual flow.

A family predisposition to the disease could be conclusive here. There is a good chance that Franny already had endometriosis before taking oral contraceptives. The likelihood is that the estrogen in the pill stimulated the growth of endometrial cells to a certain degree. And since being overweight has been connected to higher levels of estrogen, I would strongly recommend that Franny keep her weight down.

Women with Jacqui and Franny's history of endometriosis may find themselves facing a problematic option upon reaching menopause: should they have hormone replacement therapy? Such hormone therapy, in the form of estrogen supplements, is prescribed to control hot flashes, loss of vaginal elasticity, and other signs of aging related to lowering of female hormone levels. Mild endometriosis can occur as a result of estrogen replacement therapy, and this is not just the case with lifelong sufferers. Women without any disabling symptoms of the disease may find that the estrogen has activated dormant cells. Jacqui and Franny, and women who share their problem, may have to battle a recurrence of the disease when they reach menopause. Perhaps by that time, however, doctors will have found a cure that frees a woman from the disease throughout her lifetime.

Scientists seeking the organic causes of endometriosis have scrutinized genetics, chemistry of the body, the influence of stress, distress, and the tempo of a woman's life, hormonal responsibility, and even emotional attitudes. Sometimes there is great excitement in a laboratory or a doctor makes an astute observation and our knowledge of endometriosis is increased. Each quest for information brings us closer to the answer of why. Progress is being made. Until we can cite the precise components that cause endometriosis, we can work with effective methods for controlling and preventing the disease. That begins with you: your body will tell you what's wrong, but you must be able to communicate your symptoms to a doctor. For now, let's take the emphasis off *why* and learn what you can do to help yourself by understanding the disease more fully.

CHAPTER 6

What If I Have Endometriosis? What Do I Do Next?

A man in Oregon wrote to me after Elizabeth, his wife, asked him to read about endometriosis in an earlier book of mine, *Listen to Your Body*. Jonathan, a twenty-seven-year-old administrator at a large company in Texas, was searching for an answer that made sense. Elizabeth seemed to be suffering terribly, and it was getting worse. What he read about endometriosis seemed to correlate with Elizabeth's symptoms and life-style. He hoped I might assist him further.

His letter is a touching one. It is a love note for Elizabeth as well as a sad tale of all-too-common experiences with misdiagnosis and improper treatment of the "career woman's disease." It goes, in part, this way:

"I'm writing at a point of desperation in my wife's life. She has learned after five years of pain that she has endometriosis. Elizabeth has seen twenty doctors since 1982, when she began having chronic pain in her vulva following an abortion. Doctors couldn't find any condition that corresponded to her pain and either dismissed her as neurotic or prescribed creams that irritated the area.

"Then, a few months ago, a general practitioner diagnosed endometriosis based on her symptoms: painful urination, history of bad menstrual cramps, and abdominal pain. We heard that Danocrine would help over other treatments, but he insisted she take Norlutin, a synthetic progesterone, which created terrible side effects. Elizabeth then went to a top gynecologist on whom she'd pinned all her hopes. He told her that she had problems 'accepting a normal sex life' (we've been unable to make love for months because intercourse was so painful for Elizabeth) and that nothing else was wrong with her!

"I'm not a doctor, but since I read your book, I think I've unearthed every available medical journal on endometriosis. I feel pretty confident that Elizabeth has this disease and no other.

"I never would have believed how a woman can suffer and still be ignored by those with the power to heal if I had not seen it myself. This is why I'm writing a letter like this. Please give our problem your attention. We trust your opinion and hope you can answer us, no matter how briefly. What should we do next?"

Endometriosis can dramatically alter the daily rhythms of a woman's life, and Elizabeth is a good example of this. Often, intimate relationships change when *pain* becomes a demanding third party. In these cases, *coping* with the disease not only requires fortitude of spirit but needs the understanding of others.

Of the many points Jonathan raised in Elizabeth's case, the most significant was his description of two of the three symptoms (the "triad") that most typify endometriosis: *a history of bad menstrual cramps* and *dyspareunia (or painful intercourse)*. The third, *infertility,* is, in my opinion, a good probability for Elizabeth, although getting pregnant is not relevant to her now. Therefore, I believe there is enough evidence to prove that Elizabeth is suffering from endometriosis.

Although a laparoscopy, or "Band-Aid procedure," performed by a good diagnostician can help reveal the truth about Elizabeth's condition, it's a fairly good bet based on her symptoms that she has endometriosis and that a laparoscopy is not necessary in her case. As mentioned earlier, a standard suction abortion is rarely responsible for the onset of the disease. A badly performed abortion, however, may have caused some damage to the uterus. The doctor might have accidentally wrenched it in some way, tearing it slightly so that endometriotic tissue spread to the cervix and vagina. It is worth noting that the disease very rarely implants itself and grows in the vagina. However, during an internal examination a doctor can see very small brown-black ("powder burn") spots of endometriosis on the cervix.

Unless there were actual lesions or indication of infection, I would say that the pain in Elizabeth's vulva was not due to a localized problem, but radiated down from another source. Most likely, the pain originated in pelvic organs inflamed with actively growing endometriotic tissue. Such growths would also account for frequent urination, since the bladder is commonly involved in this "glue-stick" disease.

As I understand her case, I would energetically recommend for Elizabeth a program of the antihormone Danocrine, which both halts the spread of endometriotic tissue and shrinks the growths, thereby reducing or eliminating wrenching cyclical pain. Danocrine should be a help, unless it was shown that she could not tolerate it. It is not clear to me why one doctor prescribed and insisted on Norlutin, a birth control pill, since it has never been proved effective in treating endometriosis.

Beyond organic problems, I sympathize with Elizabeth's temporary collapse of effort. Who wouldn't feel despair when twenty doctors could not help her! If ever sufferers of the disease need a support system to bolster morale (husbands, lovers, friends, or other women who are experienced with the disease), it is at these times.

It is tempting to believe *exactly* what a doctor says, even if his diagnosis seems more like a weak hunch. He is the expert, after all. Blind faith does not help in the cure of the disease, however, so move on and *take charge* if you are still in pain. Find a doctor who understands endometriosis. Your health and fertility depend on this.

My guess is that the persistent frustration of poor medical care contributed further to Elizabeth's illness. Such stress—that is, negative psychological stress—is known to increase adrenal gland output, which then pumps up blood pressure, thereby increasing cholesterol levels in the blood. Negative stress tends to keep blood pressure up. Eventually, immune system barriers will break down and, combined with high blood pressure from unresolved stress, will impair healing.

I see in this letter an unmistakable lesson: this disease must be met head-on. This is why I urge women to arm themselves with knowledge of the disease's key symptoms and become more actively involved in their own health care.

Partnership of any kind, but especially partnership in health care, requires harmonious goals. You and your doctor must be able to exchange information freely and decide on the wisest course of action.

WHAT YOUR DOCTOR SHOULD KNOW:
WOMEN TELL THEIR STORIES

Annie's Story: Annie is a twenty-seven-year-old advertising copywriter. Annie wants to clear up her health problem, but she is confused about what is wrong with her. Her story starts this way: "Since I was about sixteen, I've had stabbing pain in my left side and back during my period. I was told it was part of being a woman. About a year ago, I doubled over in severe pain and had to be taken to the emergency room. I was so wiped out, they gave me a blood test to ensure that I was not bleeding internally. Ultrasound confirmed a cyst on my right ovary. The doctor said it would be reabsorbed by my body in the weeks that followed (which was later confirmed). That's all they found, yet I left the hospital in pain! I couldn't eat or sleep for the pain. I called my doctor again and he said it might be an infection, or even gonorrhea, and that I should come in for a test. How could it be a venereal disease? I've had this pain for eleven years!"

Annie's experience is one I've heard again and again. Unfortunately, a majority of doctors do not suspect endometriosis when a differential diagnosis *seemingly* confirms pelvic inflammatory disease (PID) or, in some cases, gonorrhea. Cramps, back pain, abdominal tenderness, and other symptoms tend to indicate pelvic inflammatory disease; additionally, gonorrhea left untreated creates a few symptoms that can resemble endometriosis, including abnormal bleeding and severe pelvic pain. However, there is often accompanying fever with advanced gonorrhea (pus from resulting tubal or ovarian abscesses may cause pelvic inflammation), which does not occur in cases of endometriosis. I emphasize this confusion in diagnosis because a majority of doctors suggest the possibility of infection *first*. Antibiotics, as previously noted, do not help sufferers of endometriosis.

Cysts are a common ovarian abnormality. They vary in content and can be benign or malignant. A *simple* cyst, which is a fluid-filled sac, can grow on an ovary anytime during the menstrual cycle. A *dermoid* cyst contains types of skin tissue, is more solid in character, and grows less frequently. Most ovarian cysts will disappear spontaneously after one or two menstrual cycles and are therefore not much cause for alarm. This is the type of cyst doctors thought Annie had, but such cysts tend not to cause much pain. In Annie's case, pain was severe.

Endometrial cysts, called endometriomas, grow faster than either simple cysts or dermoids and can cause more pain—the kind of pain Annie was feeling. Endometriomas are also called chocolate cysts or blood cysts, since they are filled with old blood and endometrial cells, and they are deep brown in color. An endometriotic cyst can be very large, even bigger than a grapefruit, or smaller than a pea. Interestingly, smaller cysts can cause more pain than larger ones and may make diagnosis more difficult.

Wendy's Story: Wendy, a thirty-one-year-old manager of a Florida boutique, has been married for three years. She has been trying to get pregnant but has encountered many difficulties. Wendy described her crisis: "After doing a laparoscopy on me, my doctor told me I didn't have endometriosis. He said I was okay, yet I'm in pain two weeks of every month. I want a baby, but it's hard to feel sexy when you feel so bad. Even so, I've been pregnant three times in the last two and a half years, but I have miscarried each one. What could be wrong with me?"

Wendy's plight is one many women with undiagnosed endometriosis understand all too well: pain, infertility, and no adequate explanation for their symptoms. In the past, it was felt that endometriosis in a more advanced stage prevented pregnancy because cysts and massive adhesions set up a hostile environment for conception. Most recent research into the subject, however, has revealed that a one-to-one correlation between infertility and endometriosis exists at earlier stages, too. (A chapter devoted to this will explicate further.) This research on earlier-stage endometriosis is particularly relevant to Wendy's case.

A team of doctors at the University of Kentucky Medical Center's Reproductive Endocrinology Department in Lexington concluded, in their 1985 study, that women with mild endometriosis suffered twice the number of spontaneous abortions, or miscarriage, that women with the disease at a more serious stage suffered. In examining this phenomenon, Michael Vernon, Ph.D., and his colleagues speculated that early or milder endometriotic lesions might be more "metabolically active" and produce prostaglandins, the hormones that have been implicated in the activity of endometriotic tissue. Prostaglandins might be partially responsible for infertility and miscarriage, since they cause uterine and tubal cramping, thus making conception and full-term pregnancy more difficult.

In further testing, they examined various types of implants, from very mild to serious. These implants have, in fact, been classified on a rating system to standardize their description for doctors. Devised by the American Fertility Society, this system charts and describes implants by color and degree of growth, and rates them on a scale of severity from I to IV. (See the illustration on page 66.) Implants may be red, reddish brown, dark brown, or black (also known as powder burn). The Kentucky team also discovered that the "mildest" implants produced and synthesized twice the amount of prostaglandin F that implants at an intermediary stage produced, which in turn produced more of the hormone than the powder-burn variety. (In some experi-

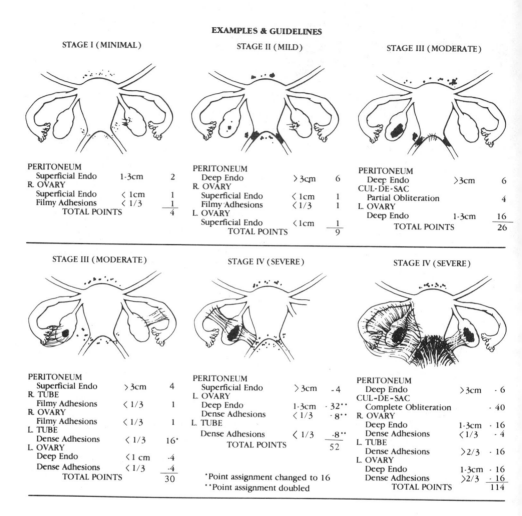

EXAMPLES & GUIDELINES

STAGE I (MINIMAL)

PERITONEUM
Superficial Endo   1-3cm   2
R. OVARY
Superficial Endo   < 1cm   1
Filmy Adhesions   < 1/3   1
     TOTAL POINTS   4

STAGE II (MILD)

PERITONEUM
Deep Endo   > 3cm   6
R. OVARY
Superficial Endo   < 1cm   1
Filmy Adhesions   < 1/3   1
L. OVARY
Superficial Endo   < 1cm   1
     TOTAL POINTS   9

STAGE III (MODERATE)

PERITONEUM
Deep Endo   > 3cm   6
CUL-DE-SAC
Partial Obliteration   4
L. OVARY
Deep Endo   1-3cm   16
     TOTAL POINTS   26

STAGE III (MODERATE)

PERITONEUM
Superficial Endo   > 3cm   4
R. TUBE
Filmy Adhesions   < 1/3   1
R. OVARY
Filmy Adhesions   < 1/3   1
L. TUBE
Dense Adhesions   < 1/3   16*
L. OVARY
Deep Endo   < 1 cm   4
Dense Adhesions   < 1/3   4
     TOTAL POINTS   30

STAGE IV (SEVERE)

PERITONEUM
Superficial Endo   > 3cm   4
L. OVARY
Deep Endo   1-3cm   32**
Dense Adhesions   < 1/3   8**
L. TUBE
Dense Adhesions   < 1/3   8**
     TOTAL POINTS   52

*Point assignment changed to 16
**Point assignment doubled

STAGE IV (SEVERE)

PERITONEUM
Deep Endo   > 3cm   6
CUL-DE-SAC
Complete Obliteration   40
R. OVARY
Deep Endo   1-3cm   16
Dense Adhesions   < 1/3   4
L. TUBE
Dense Adhesions   > 2/3   16
L. OVARY
Deep Endo   1-3cm   16
Dense Adhesions   > 2/3   16
     TOTAL POINTS   114

How would your doctor pinpoint and classify the degree of endometriosis involving your reproductive organs? These six diagrams are considered the latest definitive classification, as established by the American Fertility Society. This chart system is set up to clarify the extent of the disease by location, size, and number of endometrial growths involving the ovaries, uterus, fallopian tubes, cul-de-sac, and peritoneum. A point system is designated to each implant, depending on its *size*. For example, a 1cm (one centimeter) implant as shown in Stage 1, *Ovary* Superficial Endo (above), is equal to one point. As the doctor finds implants and determines their size, he assigns points to them, then adds up the points. As the disease spreads and the implants increase in size and severity, the points get higher and the disease is assigned a different stage number. How these stages affect a woman's fertility will be explained in chapter 12.

ments, powder-burn implants produced no such hormone.) This explains why women with minimal endometriosis sometimes experience more pain than women with massive growths. (Massive growths are simply easier to identify.)

Wendy's doctor clearly suspected endometriosis—no doubt his reason for performing a laparoscopy. That he was unable to find any *obvious* trace of the disease led to his conclusion that she was free of it. My advice to Wendy is to return to her doctor to begin a program of Danocrine to halt endometriotic growth, and to start on a diet high in complex carbohydrates and rich in B vitamins—the vitamins that are important in combating stress and favoring conception.

Christina's Story: After working for an insurance company for five years, twenty-five-year-old Christina decided to do what she'd always felt suited her best—she became a police officer. Christina leads a high-stress life, and although she experiences pelvic pain, she has been told that she does not have endometriosis. Christina tells it this way: "I've had cramping my whole life, and days of heavy bleeding, and I can't afford to be fuzzy-headed when it's a matter of life and death. My doctor says I don't have endometriosis, just cramps. My mother had a hysterectomy when she was fifty-two (two years ago) and the gynecologist told her that her abdominal organs were almost literally cemented together by endometriosis. He was amazed that her intestines weren't completely obstructed. I want to keep this disease in control and wonder if there's some way to 'track' it. If I can predict a bad day, I can be better prepared."

There are many ways to follow the symptoms of endometriosis as they seesaw through the month, but first we need to differentiate between *normal* cyclical functions—that is, menstruation—and *abnormal* conditions. Normal function includes an approximate twenty-eight-day cycle with some premenstrual pelvic pressure and bloating. Any menstrual cramps can easily be controlled with Midol or aspirin. Discomforting premenstrual symptoms will vary from person to person, sometimes including midmonth low-range pain (mittelschmerz), indicating ovulation.

Christina can increase her awareness of the disease by using a calendar, like the one that follows. (You can photocopy this calendar for your own use.) Ideally, entries should begin with the first day of menstrual bleeding, which is an absolute marker. Each day, symptoms should be listed from good to bad, as the sample below indicates for

Symptoms of endometriosis tend to follow a recurrent pattern month after month. Every woman will notice a different degree of cramping, pain (concentrated on her right side, left side, or radiating down her leg, etc.), headaches, and general malaise. To get the most from this calendar, also note when you use aspirin, over-the-counter preparations that contain ibuprofen (prostaglandin inhibitors), or tranquilizers. *Ovulation* occurs midmonth between periods, or approximately on the eleventh to fifteenth days. You may be someone who suffers from symptoms of PMS (premenstrual syndrome) approximately five days before menstruation, *coexisting* with the symptoms of endometriosis. PMS symptoms may include bloating, depression or mood swings, breast tenderness, sleep disturbances, and frequency of urination, among others. *Check off symptoms* that occur month to month on approximately the same days. Those listed below are only a sample. Add symptoms that are specific to you.

- Bleeding (light, moderate, heavy)
- Spotting
- Cramps (severe, bearable, mild)
- Leg cramps
- Backache
- Fainting
- Headache
- Dizziness

- Diarrhea
- Stabbing pain (right side, left side, stomach)
- Bloating
- Pelvic pressure
- Pain during intercourse
- Frequent urination
- Depression
- Appetite (increased, decreased)

Month _____ 19 _____

WEEK	SUNDAY	MONDAY	TUESDAY	WEDNESDAY	THURSDAY	FRIDAY	SATURDAY
1							
2							
3							
4							
5							

Notes

Month MARCH   1987

WEEK	SUNDAY	MONDAY	TUESDAY	WEDNESDAY	THURSDAY	FRIDAY	SATURDAY
1	Heavy bleeding cramps Fainted Dizziness Stayed home	Leg cramps Less bleeding Backache Confusion Diarrhea At home	Less bleeding Cramps Dizziness Back to work reluctantly	Cramps Stabbing pain in stomach Loss of appetite	Staining Minimal cramps Urinary frequency Feel washed out	Minimum staining Cramps nearly gone Slight headache	No bleeding Feel better
2	Feel good	Feel okay	Feel good again	Feel good	Slight abdominal pain	Pressure and pain on left side Slight staining	Pain after intercourse Some bleeding Dizzy
3	Feel better Slight staining	Feel good	Feel good Slight pain after intercourse	Feel good	Feel okay	Slight headache	Feel good
4	Feel good No pain after intercourse	Feel good	Feel good	Bloating Abdominal pressure	Very hungry Intermittent abdominal pain Pelvic pain	Spotting	Increased pelvic pressure and pain Painful intercourse
5	Fainted Severe abdominal pain	Heavy bleeding Frequent urination Bad cramps	Less bleeding cramps and pain helped with ibuprofen				

Notes

Christina. Over a two-month period, it will become clear when the side effects of high levels of prostaglandins are the most virulent. Those effects may include severe cramps, fainting, diarrhea, and pounding headache. There are also cases in which endometriotic tissue growing on the fallopian tubes causes a special dysfunction: during ovulation, the fallopian tube "misfires" and cannot draw in all the fluid surrounding the egg. Some of this fluid drops into the abdomen, causing tremendous pain. Furthermore, some women will experience psychological symptoms of premenstrual syndrome (PMS) along with the more physically debilitating problems associated with endometriosis.

Keeping a chart of her symptoms is vital for helping a woman and her doctor assess the severity of the disease and select an appropriate treatment.

Sandra's Story: Sandra is a nineteen-year-old Texas native, a student of oceanography at a West Coast college. Sandra had surgery when she was fourteen years old—an ovarian cyst had burst. She had been enduring moderately unpleasant menstrual cramps until a year before she consulted me, when they increased in severity. Sandra reports: "I thought I was okay, but I've begun to bleed abnormally. I have terrible pain in my right side, and my doctor now tells me that my ovary is very enlarged and he thinks I may have endometriosis. He wants to put me into the hospital for a laparoscopy. The idea of surgery scares me. What does this procedure *really* involve?"

Judging from Sandra's history of ovarian problems, I would certainly want to be sure that she is suffering from endometriosis, and not another disorder. There is a good chance that a sonogram and laparoscopy would clarify the diagnosis of her condition.

LAPAROSCOPY:
ONE WAY TO DIAGNOSE ENDOMETRIOSIS

Laparoscopy is a fairly simple procedure that yields excellent results when done correctly.

When the modern and very versatile laparoscope was invented in Sweden about twenty years ago, it was the culmination of a long medical quest to look into and observe the living human body. It is fiber optics, or cold light, that made the laparoscope possible and practical to make. The laparoscope is a long rigid tube equipped with thin glass fibers (along which light travels to "spotlight" organs) and a periscopelike attachment that allows doctors to see into the pelvis and abdomen. Lightweight and flexible (it can be maneuvered into various positions), the laparoscope not only makes it possible to see into the abdominal cavity but can also be used along with surgical instruments, if necessary, for further medical procedures. Therefore, laparoscopy—the technique that employs the tool—can be performed for either a diagnostic or a therapeutic procedure. (See the illustration below.)

The most frequent candidates for laparoscopy are women with fertility problems, but the number of women who are suspected of having endometriosis and are undergoing the technique to confirm it is growing apace. Laparoscopy, it has been found, benefits women with either problem (or both) in this way: since the technique allows a

LAPAROSCOPY

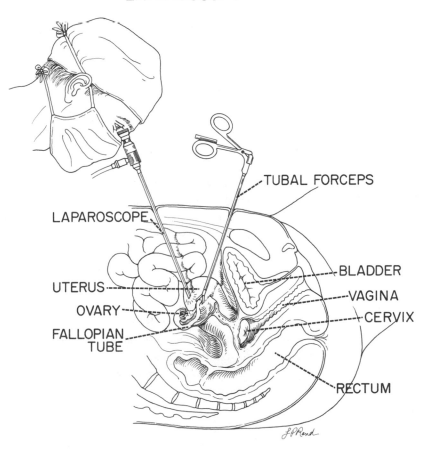

71

visual inspection of pelvic organs and subsequent diagnosis, it can avert major surgery. For patients with persistently *misdiagnosed* and *undiagnosed* pelvic pain, it may finally provide an answer. Doctors can look for signs of endometriosis in its varying stages—from a reddened inflamed appearance of organs to the existence of pepper spots to greater gluelike adhesions to more massive chocolate cysts and tumors. Laparoscopy allows the sighting of such conditions, but remember, it *is* surgery, though on a lesser scale.

Currently, laparoscopy, familiarly called the Band-Aid procedure, is considered by most doctors to be the only absolute method of detection for endometriosis. Would that it were absolute! As it turns out, *laparoscopy is only as good as the practitioner doing the viewing and diagnosing.* Endometriosis is sometimes difficult to identify. Endometriosis that is growing on the ligaments behind the uterus or hidden inside tissue can be difficult to spot. To locate such growths, a doctor needs skill and dexterity. The scope must be positioned well below the uterus to catch sight of hard-to-see implants.

Unfortunately, some physicians either are inexperienced or may not fully understand the procedure or the female anatomy, or both. Because of these shortcomings, a number of complications can occur during laparoscopy. If it is not conducted under proper sterile techniques, the procedure can lead to abdominal and pelvic infections. Internal bleeding is a possibility from an incorrectly placed laparoscope; the device can lacerate, perforate, or traumatize the organs. Laparoscopy can cause serious problems like these in the hands of an unskilled physician. Then again, he may be knowledgeable enough about the procedure itself, but lacking as a diagnostician.

Cases of women undergoing this procedure and being told they are free of the disease when, in fact, they are *not* are not uncommon. One reason, as mentioned, is the surgeon's skill in detecting it. Another is that the endometriosis may be microscopic and not visible to the eye. This means that evidence of the disease may not be revealed with laparoscopy, although it exists. Otherwise, the disease is officially described at four different stages of severity (I, II, III, and IV), as recently classified by the American Fertility Society (see the illustration on page 66). Sharon's story, which I will share with you in a moment, demonstrates the course of such aforementioned misdiagnoses, not once but three times. First, let's get a better sense of the procedure and see how and why it works.

How Laparoscopies Are Performed

Laparoscopies are most often conducted at a hospital or clinic where the patient normally is put under general anesthesia. I believe general anesthesia is the best agent for women undergoing laparoscopies, although a number of patients may benefit from local anesthesia along with a common analgesic like Demerol or Valium, the alternate choice sometimes preferred by doctors. Surgery begins with an incision that is made either in the navel or directly below it. My preference is to make a horizontal incision inside the navel, placed about a quarter of an inch across its deepest inner recess. Such incisions, when healed, form no visible scar. Sometimes a second incision may be made—this one just above the pubic bone—to insert instruments which can help get a better view of the lower abdomen. A small peritoneal needle is then inserted through the navel into the abdomen, into which is pumped four liters of carbon dioxide (CO_2) gas. (Carbon dioxide is preferred over oxygen because it is safer—nonexplosive and easily absorbable. The biggest problem with oxygen is that it is flammable; sometimes doctors use lasers and electrocautery during this procedure, and any oxygen will cause burns in the abdomen.) After the gas has properly inflated the abdomen, the laparoscope is inserted into the incision.

The doctor wants to get the best and most unobstructed view of the pelvic organs. To do that, he adjusts his patient's position. The carbon dioxide has already helped separate the organs, so they can be seen more clearly. Now he will tip the patient so her head is tilted downward, causing the bowel to float upward toward the chest. This position provides him with the required unobstructed view of the pelvic organs, which are set slightly afloat in the distended abdomen.

The laparoscope provides a viewing lens and a light—much like a flashlight shining through a buttonhole. When the laparoscope is in place, the doctor looks through it, moving it within its range of flexibility to view his patient's internal organs. He may also introduce other instruments through it either to move aside an organ that may block a view or to perform minor surgery.

If a doctor notices any abnormality—of the ovaries, for example—he is able to insert a needle through the hollow laparoscope and aspirate, or remove, sample cells from this organ for a biopsy. A tissue biopsy is the best way to diagnose endometriosis, but the process can be tricky. The endometrial implant may be on a part of an organ that is difficult to get to, or the implant may be so small that it is difficult to get a proper sample. There are occasions, too, where taking a tissue sample for a biopsy is successful, but there may be some confusion about the *results* of the biopsy. I have biopsied lumps that come back positive for endometriosis after patients had been told they did not have the disease. This might have happened either because the doctor did not do a biopsy during laparoscopy or because he did not know how to identify endometriosis. I have seen remarkable cases in which my patient's symptoms were clear-cut profiles of endometriosis even though the laparoscopy informed me of *no* organic signs but a biopsy of tissue came back positive.

Since the fallopian tubes are delicate structures, the doctor will check them for adhesions, to see if they have narrowed or are

WHEN IS LAPAROSCOPY NECESSARY AND WHEN IS IT UNNECESSARY?

Laparoscopy is one of the best diagnostic tools for determining the existence and extent of pelvic endometriosis, but remember: laparoscopy is a surgical procedure. It may not be *major* abdominal surgery, but it is still an invasive operation.

Laparoscopy can be agreed to under the following circumstances:

• Cases in which the doctor cannot determine if a tender pelvic mass is caused by pelvic inflammatory disease (PID), an ectopic pregnancy, pelvic endometriosis, or even appendicitis.

• Women who have pelvic masses or ovarian cysts that persist through a few menstrual cycles and who *do not have* characteristically clinical symptoms of endometriosis. These signs are severe menstrual cramps, pain during intercourse, pain during ovulation, and increasing pelvic pain prior to menstruation. If the nature of the cysts cannot first be determined by a pelvic sonogram, laparoscopy is indicated to confirm endometriosis and to exclude the presence of fibroid tumors, ovarian cysts, ovarian cancer, or any other abnormality.

• Women who *do have* clinical signs of endometriosis and who have not improved significantly after being treated with Danocrine for up to six months.

• Women who *do have* clinical signs of endometriosis and are being treated with Danocrine or other medication but who then develop a pelvic mass which *increases* in size during such treatment. Any increase of the growth of a mass can be a warning sign of malignancy.

• Women who do not become pregnant after several months of attempting conception, especially those women with suspected or verified cases of endometriosis. A laparoscopy may be indicated to determine the causes of infertility after they have been unsuccessfully treated with fertility drugs and evaluated with all available fertility tests, such as hormone analysis, an X ray of the uterus and tubes or hysterosalpingogram, sperm analysis, and so on.

• A "second-look" procedure for women who have been cured of endometriosis, who have experienced complete remission of the disease, but who subsequently develop a mass or tumor whose nature cannot be determined other than by laparoscopy.

There are also occasions when laparoscopy is *unnecessary.* This procedure is *not* indicated in the following cases:

• Women who *do have* early clinical signs of endometriosis and who experience pelvic tenderness and pain during an internal examination but whose doctors do not feel any cysts or enlarged pelvic masses. Endometriosis in its mildest and earliest stages does not result in cysts large enough for doctors to palpate. Furthermore, the laparoscopist could not see microscopic endometriosis, or he might diagnose it as an inflammatory condition.

• Women whose endometriosis at its earliest stages either has been *un*diagnosed or *mis*diagnosed and who have already gone to the expense of a laparoscopy that failed to diagnose the disease. If all their symptoms clearly add up to the clinical signs of endometriosis, these women should be treated with an approved medication such as Danocrine for three to six months to control the disease.

• Women with proven endometriosis who have been successfully treated with Danocrine in the past and are now experiencing the same recurring clinical symptoms and whose doctors confirm the same pelvic findings. Instead of a laparoscopy, these women can again be given approved medication such as Danocrine to control the disease.

obstructed, a possible result of endometriosis, or if there are any ravaging effects of previous conditions. At this point during the procedure, he can inject a blue dye, which will define the condition of the tubes and reveal whether or not they are open. One result of pelvic inflammatory disease, for example, is that the fimbriated (fingerlike) ends of the tubes clump together and lose their ability to transport the egg from the ovary to the tube, where conception normally takes place. A number of other procedures that may involve the fallopian tubes are available, such as testing for obstructions by injecting dyes and tracing their course, otherwise known as a hysterosalpingogram, which will be discussed in full very shortly.

When the laparoscopy is over, the carbon dioxide gas is let out, the abdomen deflates, and the small incision is either sewn or stapled closed and covered with a Band-Aid—hence the procedure's sobriquet. There may be a few aftereffects from the surgery, such as slight nausea, difficulty urinating, and sometimes pain in the shoulders, but these episodes are brief. Shoulder pain, should it occur, is a result of the tilted position during the operation and the pressure of the CO_2 gas against the diaphragm. This pressure irritates nerves and pain radiates up to the shoulders. Most women, however, are able to return

---

WHO SHOULD NOT HAVE A LAPAROSCOPY?

Although the procedure is a generally safe one, some women should definitely avoid laparoscopy:

• Obese women are not good candidates for laparoscopy. The amount of body fat makes it difficult for the doctor to position the instrument correctly.

• Women with a history of extensive abdominal surgery are at greater risk for complications. This is because pelvic adhesions (scar tissue) may exist as a result of previous operations. The combination of endometrial growths *and* adhesions on the bowel can bind it down, making surgery complicated and bowel perforation possible. If the bowel is perforated when a laparoscope is inserted, a chain of needless problems can arise, including serious infection.

• Women with cardiovascular disease and/or high blood pressure are also at greater risk and should not agree to this procedure.

---

home the following day without any problem. For about a week or two, abdominal soreness or a dull pain may be bothersome, but in general, the only sign of surgery should be a tiny unseen scar in the navel, and sex is safely resumed about a week after surgery.

Laparoscopy and the Doctor's Point of View

Typically, a gynecologist knows that a laparoscopy is indicated when his patient's complaints of pelvic pain persist for at least six months and he finds that she is not responding to conservative treatment, such as painkillers, or to a regimen of antibiotics (if he found signs of infection). He will need to reevaluate her case at this point: did she have endometriosis at the time of her first visit to his office? Let's assume that the doctor isn't sure and now she is back at his office, having followed all his instructions. She is not better, but worse, valiantly struggling with her pain and seeking relief. Her doctor suggests laparoscopy, since it may be endometriosis that's causing her symptoms. He assures her that even if it is not, the procedure may help reveal any of several other conditions, such as acute ovarian cysts or even an ectopic pregnancy.

It is my feeling that a good diagnostician should be about 95 percent sure that his patient has endometriosis just by taking a very detailed medical history and listening to her progression of symptoms. A follow-up laparoscopy, when indicated, could then confirm the diagnosis. I have discovered, however, that there is another side to the issue: many women have had unfortunate experiences not only with misdiagnosis at the time of their initial visit but with laparoscopy as well. As the patient, you should be aware of what steps your doctor is taking before he recommends a laparoscopy:

• If the doctor believes you have an infection, he should have taken a culture to prove that point.

• If the doctor suggests that you have a pelvic cyst or tumor, it should have been confirmed first with a pelvic ultrasound.

• If you are not responding to any treatment the doctor prescribes based on his findings, you should then be free and able to openly discuss with him (1) how you feel and (2) what other diagnostic and therapeutic steps could be taken.

• If he first retests you for infections, cysts, and tumors and all the tests are negative once again, a laparoscopy might then be called for.

What happens when a woman willingly undergoes this procedure again and again and is either diagnosed correctly or incorrectly, and either way, the disease is mismanaged? Sharon, a twenty-six-year-old secretary at a law firm in New Mexico, sent me a letter describing her trials with serial laparoscopies. I think this is important reading if you are about to have a laparoscopy, and, if you have experienced a similar situation, you will understand Sharon's frustration.

Sharon's Story: Four Laparoscopies— "Does Anyone Know What's Wrong with Me?"

"Looking back on a five-year problem that had me hospitalized four times for laparoscopies, I find it shocking that my now-diagnosed endometriosis could have been overlooked by a count of *ten out of twelve* doctors! What is amazing is that the *first* laparoscopy showed endometriosis, and some of the adhesions were cauterized at that time. Unfortunately, the doctor who said it was endometriosis attributed the adhesions to an infection, even though a blood test showed no such thing.

"Four months later, the pain started again and the doctor did a second laparoscopy. His words were 'no findings,' meaning that he couldn't *see* the endometriosis, not necessarily that it wasn't there. I went to another doctor, this time traveling to a big medical center in the Midwest, and he had vague explanations about my pain after giving me a third laparoscopy. For about five months, I started to improve by some miracle. I was taking pain pills until last summer and then the crash came. The pain was so intense I couldn't stand up. I was put on antibiotics again. The doctor said my case was 'too peculiar' and he increased the dosage of painkillers.

"A cousin sent me to her doctor. He actually listened to all of my symptoms (no one else really heard them when I recounted them) and he diagnosed endometriosis, but sent me to *another* doctor to have a fourth laparoscopy to be sure. It showed endometriosis, with one big implant near my left tube and another two implants on my right ovary.

"What is really disturbing to me is that all these doctors were highly recommended. The third doctor even told me that if the second doctor found nothing after a laparoscopy, then nothing was there! The doctor who gave me the fourth laparoscopy put me on Danocrine for four days, but I had such bad reactions to the drug that he decided birth control pills would be better. I was still in pain after taking these pills, so he changed the brand. Now he wants to do a *fifth* laparoscopy 'to get an objective view of the pain,' and if that's not enough, he wants to perform a laparotomy!"

Sharon's chance for treatment and possible cure was sabotaged by her first doctor's misdiagnosis. Sadly, it set her on an unwitting course that would be repeated again and again with other doctors. As it happened, the first laparoscopy revealed adhesions—fibrous bands that can bind organs. Adhesions are unrelated to pelvic infections, but they do signal the possible presence of endometriosis.

Endometriosis can sometimes be detected during a pelvic examination if the masses are large enough to be felt. In Sharon's case, the "hidden disease" had infiltrated pelvic tissue and was detectable with the aid of a laparoscope. Since its nature is also to implant itself on organs and go unseen, endometriosis can be missed by doctors who are not familiar with identifying and treating the disease. This happened to her three times.

The Difference Between Laparoscopy and Laparotomy

Will laparotomy help Sharon?

Unlike laparoscopy, which is, in a way, exploratory surgery, laparotomy is a much more serious consideration, and should not be thought of as routine. Exploratory laparotomy is a major surgical procedure. The doctor makes a horizontal or vertical incision in the abdomen in order to explore the abdominal cavity for any abnormality or to remove tumors or cysts. This procedure is not used routinely as a diagnostic tool, but if a woman has a large pelvic cyst or mass that needs to be removed, a laparotomy might be indicated and might help treat the patient. Surprisingly, endometriosis often is discovered when something else is suggested, such as pelvic infection or pelvic tumors.

My recommendation to Sharon was to save her money and avoid any doctor who sought to check her into the hospital to do more surgical procedures with promises of accurate diagnosis.

Sharon's instincts about her condition were right from the start; she would have been better off searching for a specialist in endometriosis. Specialists are a good bet because they have experience in treating endometriosis on a regular basis, frequently are involved in research on the disease, and are more skilled with the laparoscope.

CULDOSCOPY: ANOTHER VIEW

Before laparoscopy, culdoscopy had a reputation as being a good diagnostic aid for women who were suffering from endometriosis or infertility. Laparoscopy has gained favor as the *better* tool for two reasons: the use of carbon dioxide allows a clearer view of abdominal organs (culdoscopy uses no gas), and a greater number of other techniques are possible during the procedure. Culdoscopy has a few shortcomings, but is an accepted diagnostic procedure and may still be used from time to time by practitioners who are, it is hoped, experienced at it.

Culdoscopy can be a somewhat tricky procedure, requiring experience and skill. A small incision is made in the vaginal wall into the abdominal cavity and a periscopelike instrument is inserted through it, offering a view of the uterus, ovaries, and the fallopian tubes. To make that incision, a woman must remain in a slightly awkward position that requires some of her conscious control and cooperation. Because of this positioning, she is not put under general anesthesia. (See illustration.)

CULDOSCOPY

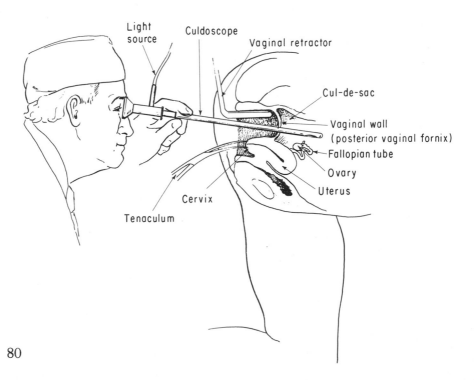

80

How Culdoscopy Is Done

Doctors prefer to do culdoscopies in a hospital with patients put under local anesthesia. Before the culdoscope can be inserted properly, the woman is positioned on the table in a kneeling position, leaning forward with her bottom higher than her chest and her head resting on her arm. Before the procedure, the vagina is washed to the point of sterilization. This is the first possible snag of culdoscopy. Since complete vaginal sterilization is impossible, there is an inherent risk of infection and doctors must proceed cautiously. After she is covered with a sterile drape, the doctor administers a spinal or epidural anesthetic, or the woman can be given a painkiller like Demerol as well. A specialized speculum is then inserted into the vagina to permit a better view of the cervix. About now, a local anesthetic is injected into the vagina and a small probe inserted blindly through the vaginal wall. When the probe is in place, a larger probe containing the culdoscope is inserted. Looking through the culdoscope, the doctor can inspect the area just behind the uterus, the ovaries, and the tubes. Since the intestines tend to fall forward while in this kneeling position, the doctor has a less obstructed view to check for any abnormality in the area.

As with laparoscopy, there is a range of therapeutic procedures, though more limited, that may be performed while the culdoscope is in place. Fine operating instruments may be inserted through it for use in minor operations, the most common of which are tubal sterilization and the removal of small adhesions.

Aftereffects of culdoscopy are usually not troublesome. If you are scheduled for one, expect minimal pelvic pain for a day or two after surgery. Doctors will advise abstinence from intercourse for three or four weeks or until complete healing has occurred. Unlike laparoscopy, which is not as debilitating, culdoscopy will require rest at home for a week or two and avoidance of stress-filled work schedules.

OTHER DIAGNOSTIC PROCEDURES FOR DETECTING ENDOMETRIOSIS

Ultrasound

Nature provided the whale and the bat with the miracle of an innate sonar system. Scientists studied the process, pretty much duplicating it for its original technological intent—wartime vigilance. During

World War II, navy submarines negotiated their way through deepest waters using sonar to detect the location of enemy vessels unseen by periscopic sighting.

Sonar is the simple process of bouncing high-frequency acoustical vibrations off solid masses. The waves then bounce back in echo patterns that appear as a picture on a specially devised screen. Sonar is the mother of sonography, or ultrasonography, known familiarly as ultrasound—a relatively new and popular diagnostic technique, gaining ever increasing acceptance for confirmation of pelvic abnormalities. It is a convenient way to diagnose both pelvic masses and fetal size (sometimes, too, the sex of the unborn child) during pregnancy. Doctors are choosing sonography over X rays for a variety of diagnoses, especially since ultrasound is completely harmless to the body.

When these high-frequency sounds are projected into the body, the reflected "echo" on the screen indicates the size and location of a tumor. Doctors can freeze the picture of a growth on the screen and measure it. The technique is especially useful in locating uterine fibroids and ovarian cysts, although occasionally, there is difficulty in sonographic diagnosis in defining the precise location of a tumor—is it growing on the side of the uterus or on the ovary? Since ovarian tumors are a more serious matter than uterine masses, laparoscopy might be necessary if sonography proves ineffective as a confirming diagnostic tool.

As with laparoscopy, sonography facilitates an accurate diagnosis when pelvic organs are lifted from view. The "lifting" here is done not with gas, but with water. That is, women prepare for ultrasound testing before coming to the doctor's office by drinking six to eight glasses of water, thus filling their bladders. The amply filled bladder moves organs up just enough so that the doctor can see the uterus and ovaries more clearly. A practiced ultrasonographer can usually detect a cyst and identify its type (and its contents) by the echo pattern on the screen and determine if the cyst is endometriotic in nature.

Ultrasound has its benefits, but in my opinion, this technique cannot pick up endometriosis in its early stages, when many women really need help in managing the disease and when it is most adroitly treated.

X Rays

"My doctor thinks I'm almost recovered from endometriosis," a thirty-year-old woman from Indiana wrote to me, "and I wonder. I've been trying to get pregnant for a year and a half, but have had no luck so far. My gynecologist told me that he suspects my tubes may be blocked from the endometriosis. He wants to X ray them. Isn't this dangerous? I want a baby, but I'm afraid of all this radiation."

Diana's query is one that I commonly hear from women who are recommended for special work-ups when infertility is involved. X rays should be used advisedly and infrequently, but they can be instrumental in deciding the degree of tubal damage.

Abdominal X rays will pick up only large tumors or hard masses, because these will form a shadow on the exposed film. Since endometriosis is soft tissue, it will not show up on these *standard* X rays. However, a hysterosalpingogram, or X ray of the uterus, used along with an injection of dye, has aided doctors in making an accurate diagnosis. The amount of radiation from a hysterosalpingogram is very low.

If Diana decides to go ahead with this X ray, she will find it pain-free. The procedure is simple. The test is performed while a woman is resting on an examining table. The doctor inserts a speculum into the vagina and the cervix is steadied with a special clamp. A small hollow tube, or cannula, is placed inside the cervical canal and will serve as the conduit for the injected dye. When the dye enters the uterine cavity, it is seen on a fluoroscope screen, and the doctor simultaneously takes an X ray. (If you refer to the illustration below, you can see that the dye has pushed into the uterine cavity, which appears to be normal. The right fallopian tube is open, indicated by dye spilling from the tube. The left tube is closed and damaged as a result of endometriosis; the dye has collected there and does not spill out into the pelvic cavity.)

Normally, the uterine cavity is small and triangular. If it is enlarged or if there is certain "intravasation"—that is, the dye falls into small pockets in the wall of the uterus—these signs might indicate a condition called endometriosis interna, or adenomyosis. Confined to the inside wall of the uterus and weakening it, adenomyosis can coexist with endometrial implants *outside* the uterus, or it may exist alone. Adenomyosis creates heavier menstrual flow and is responsible, in part, for continuous pain.

Sometimes, endometrial implants stick on the outside of the fallopian tubes, causing them to narrow. This X ray will outline the tubes

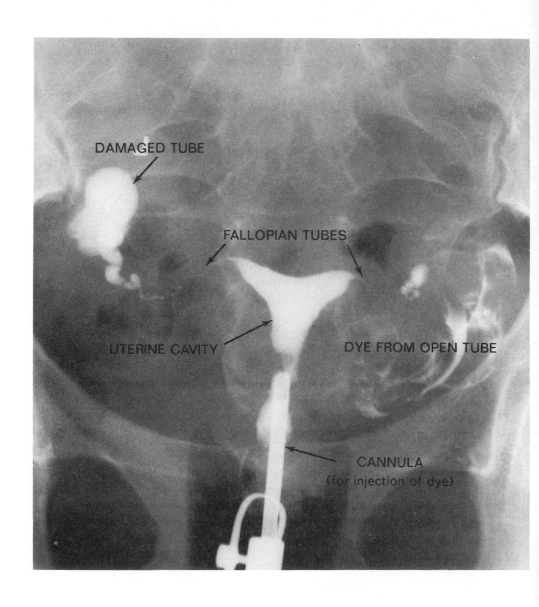

to reveal whether or not they are open, since the dye will be pushed through the hair-thin fallopian tubes. A healthy tube shows up with the dye already expelled and spilling toward the ovary and bowel. The circumstances are different when the tube is damaged. The dye won't escape, but will be trapped within one of its fimbriae, the fingerlike ends of fallopian tubes. Chances of pregnancy are nearly impossible with such a damaged tube.

Recall for a moment Sampson's theory. It proposed that the fallopian tubes were conduits for endometrial fragments during retrograde menstruation. The fallopian tube may be first to come in contact with the endometrial fragments outside the uterine cavity. Surprisingly, however, endometriosis is rarely found in the tubes. When there are endometrial implants *on* the tubes, they can be recognized by their characteristic dark blue color. In advanced cases, implants may penetrate deep into the wall of the tube, forming dense adhesions with the surrounding organs.

Tubal problems are often the cause of infertility, although it is not always endometriosis causing the problem, as it is in Diana's case. But we'll take a closer look at what happens when endometriosis affects fertility and what can be done to alleviate this in chapter 12.

FINDING BLADDER- AND KIDNEY-RELATED ENDOMETRIOSIS

"I feel like someone opened an umbrella in my bladder," one woman from Wisconsin wrote vividly in a letter to me. "I've been to a urologist five times and he gives me antibiotics, but nothing helps. For five or six days a month, all I do is go to the bathroom. It's worse when I have my period. Then I have blood in my urine, on top of all the pain. What's really wrong with me?"

Many women share Peggy's problem. They come to their doctors complaining of bladder pain, or of the sensation of needing to urinate frequently. Many of these women are suffering from endometriosis, but they are diagnosed as having bladder infections unrelated to the "career woman's disease." Endometrial tissue can implant itself on the bladder and find its way to the kidneys, where it may become a cause of future problems. The intravenous pyelogram (IVP), which is a radiographic visualization of the kidneys, can offer some clues.

In this test, dye is injected into a vein and the dye travels to the kidneys. Under X ray, these outlined organs are picked up. Cases exist in which endometriosis has invaded the kidney and leaves telltale indentations. However, even these indentations do not always con-

COMPARISON OF DIAGNOSTIC TECHNIQUES FOR ENDOMETRIOSIS

Procedure	Indication for test	Type
Laparoscopy	Pelvic tumors Pelvic mass Clinical symptoms of endometriosis	Invasive surgery
Culdoscopy	Pelvic tumors Pelvic mass Clinical symptoms of endometriosis	Invasive surgery
Pelvic sonogram	Tumors Cysts	Noninvasive procedure
Hysterosal- pingogram	Infertility Adenomyosis (often in combination with heavy bleeding)	Invasive procedure
Intravenous pyelogram	Bladder pain Tenderness around kidneys	Invasive procedure
Cystoscopy	Blood in urine Burning sensation w/ urination	Invasive procedure
Barium enema	Endometriosis in the cul-de- sac	Invasive procedure

Prediagnostic Preparation	Procedure Reveals	Postdiagnostic Care
Blood tests Electrocardiogram Fasting 6 hours before surgery	Pelvic endometriosis Pelvic adhesions Tubal patency Uterine tumors Pelvic cysts	Brief hospital stay (a few hours or overnight) Antibiotics for 5–7 days Rest at home for several days
Blood tests Electrocardiogram Fasting 6 hours before surgery	Pelvic endometriosis Pelvic adhesions Tubal patency Uterine tumors Pelvic cysts	Brief hospital stay Antibiotics for 5–7 days Rest at home for several days
None	Pelvic tumors Pelvic cysts	None
None	Tubal abnormalities Uterine abnormalities	None with no signs of infection Antibiotics with signs of infection
None	Kidney infections Endometriosis	Antibiotics with signs of infection
None	Blockage of the urethra	Medication if indicated
None	Endometriosis	None

stitute a diagnosis of endometriosis. A biopsy of tissue around the kidney is required in order to make a definitive evaluation.

Cystoscopy is another technique used to explore urinary tract dysfunction. It employs an instrument called the cystoscope, which is inserted into the urethra, making it possible to view the bladder. As with the laparoscope, the cystoscope has a built-in light source that facilitates viewing (or photographing the area) and is so constructed that doctors may take tissue biopsies at the same time.

DETERMINING ENDOMETRIOSIS IN THE BOWEL AREA

Finding endometriosis in the cul-de-sac is often a difficult task, even after laparoscopy. When endometriosis spreads through the pelvic cavity, an affected bladder may be pushed backward toward the bowel, pressing on it. A barium enema, introduced into the bowel to make the bowel sensitized to radiation, allows any growths or deformities in the intestines to show up under the scrutiny of X rays. It is not unusual for doctors to give patients this procedure twice: once early in the cycle, and a second time during menstruation to detect any actual changes.

Diagnosing endometriosis is primarily a medical matter, but it is a personal one, too. Cure requires cooperation. The more information a doctor has, the better your chances for correct treatment. Conquer endometriosis with good sense: Pay attention to your symptoms and keep a log of them. Examine your family history for unmistakable connections to the condition, especially severe menstrual cramps. Be informed about the disease and its diagnostic tools, and *tell your doctor everything related to the condition.* Do not submit to surgery without a second or third opinion, and be sure the opinions you get are not from doctors who are affiliated with the first doctor you see. Doctors who practice together or refer you to a physician of their choice may tend to think alike. This does not imply they are mistaken in their judgments; you just want to ensure a fresh point of view. Remember, today endometriosis can be diagnosed without a laparoscopy. *Your* participation in conquering endometriosis can make all the difference!

CHAPTER 7

Managing Stress (and Staying off the Emotional Roller Coaster)

WHAT can *I* do to prevent endometriosis?"

When I hear a woman ask this question, I feel assured that her chances of combating the disease are greatly improved. This statement tells me she is *actively participating in her health care,* and as a doctor, I know what this can mean in terms of cure. Although endometriosis is rarely life-threatening, it affects life on two very critical levels—well-being and fertility. I can do what I know to help sufferers in a medical context, but the women I treat also have the power to make some changes in their condition. They are often surprised by the differences *they* can make in ending the misery of endometriosis.

Taking charge of the disease involves change. There is no getting away from it. It requires a real willingness to invest in yourself and alter some daily routines and ways of thinking about the disease, as follows.

• *Build a support system.* This begins with finding a doctor who understands endometriosis and how it has affected you in particular. There is no use in convincing skeptical practitioners that you are suffering from a real condition if they persist in believing that your symptoms are psychosomatic. Use the guidelines provided in chapter 2 to find a doctor who takes this illness seriously.

Discuss your condition with family members and friends in a calm and factual manner. Explain what you have learned about the disease and why you are feeling the way you do. Severe menstrual cramping attributed to prostaglandin levels, painful intercourse, and mood swings due to hormone fluctuations are real factors in the disease. Now that your loved ones know it's not "in your head," ask for their help in getting you through any especially difficult time. If you feel you need pyschological counseling either alone or in family therapy to help sort out your feelings about the impact of the condition on you and on others, seek help now.

The "career woman's disease" touches the lives of millions of women who must deal with their condition and continue to work efficiently. This can be a problem. Many employers are not interested in hearing that employees suffer from chronic disorders such as endometriosis. As with sufferers of PMS, women with endometriosis may be assumed to be overly self-indulgent during menstruation. It has been estimated that 140 million work hours are lost each year to the symptoms of endometriosis, a fact that the business world cannot ignore.

Yet, they do. Now it is up to you. Your wisest strategy is to be consistently reasonable at work and prudent about whom you inform of your condition. Although your impulse may be to educate your employers and coworkers, many of whom may have the disease or know others who might, not everyone may be sympathetic to you. There are two schools of thought about discussing this disease and its effect on women, and doing so on the job. Some avoid public disclosure, feeling it is best to be discreet. They are concerned that knowledge of their condition may be used against them, that is, used as a reason to hold them back from greater responsibility and promotions.

Other women feel that having endometriosis is not a stigmatizing factor and that a calm, honest, and educational approach will not hinder their career advancement. These women are bolder about their approach to the disease. They may disseminate information about endometriosis, or post notices of discussion groups to alert women to what they can do for themselves and for others, too. Knowing they do not have to keep silent about their condition and finding even one other woman at work who shares their problem gives them a psychological boost and an important sense of supportiveness. The action you do or do not take at work will depend entirely on the kind of job you have and the general tone of your workplace. You will know best what to do in this case.

• *Believe you can make a difference.* You will learn what you can do to alter your condition within these pages, but you must believe, in your heart, that you can do it. Then you have to take the first step. Beginnings can seem formidable and the goal may seem far away. Keep up your energy and motivation to reach the goal of offsetting the symptoms of endometriosis, reducing the pain, and, possibly, curing the disease and preventing its recurrence. This is challenging, but it can be done by taking one step at a time.

• *Change your diet.* Endometriosis responds so well to dietary changes that I feel it must be part of standard treatment, along with medication, as indicated, for each woman. The endometriosis recovery diet follows shortly. It is based on evidence that certain foods, vitamins, and minerals affect both pain from menstrual cramping and hormone levels. The diet concentrates on putting your body in balance nutritionally and reducing pain the natural way. Put very simply, it requires you to cut down on sugar, salt, and fat and increase your intake of complex carbohydrates, certain vitamins, and fiber.

Studies show that obesity promotes higher estrogen levels, which increase the chances of endometriotic cysts. Women on vegetarian diets have higher levels of estrogen and cholesterol in their stool than meat-eaters. Essentially, all the fiber they are eating helps eliminate excess estrogen and cholesterol from their bodies. This is one reason why you need fiber.

• *Reduce stress.* Stress-related accidents and illnesses account for about three-fourths of the time lost on the job. Why does this happen? Stress attacks start a domino effect in the body. Stress is far more than a pyschological irritant. During hard stress, the lymph glands shrink; the cortisone level is raised as the adrenal glands release more of this hormone and impair immune system functioning; blood pressure rises; the heart works harder; and the body, in sum, is left open to infection or stress-related disease.

There is much dispute about stress's affecting or creating endometriosis. Some see the disease as a combination of known and unknown factors, all of them within the body itself—whether it is genetic predisposition or links to hormone production. These people, many of them sufferers of endometriosis, do not believe that stress has any real bearing on the condition, arguing that this places too much responsibility and "guilt" on the patient. Others, like myself, believe that this disease is connected in some way to the effects of counterproductive stress, such as fatigue, overwork, disruptive environments, discord among family members or friends, worry about money, career, love, and security for the future.

Dr. Christiane Northrup, an obstetrician and gynecologist and cofounder of a group practice, Women to Women, in Yarmouth, Maine, concurs. "I almost never see a patient with endometriosis who does not have a number of adverse factors in her life, which *may* have affected the onset or progress of the disease," she told me. As a woman doctor treating women, she says, "I feel strongly that stress is most definitely a component."

Dr. Northrup thinks it is helpful for women to "rethink their goals" and do some "inner searching." What does she mean? "Modern women want their lives to be an organic whole," she said. "Ideally, this means home life is consistent with work life, rather like an *intermeshed flowing whole*. I think it's common for working women to be hard on themselves and add the self-induced pressures of wanting that harmony and balance, myself included.

"Women have to realize that they must be responsible for their health. It's urgent that we abandon a helplessness in our way of thinking, take charge of the disease, and ask, 'Why do I have this and what can *I* do about it now?' I suggest women make the changes as they can and try not to let 'absolutes' such as a genetic predisposition to endometriosis lock them into feeling at the mercy of the disease."

STRESS-REDUCTION TIPS

Not everything in life has the same measure of importance. The day has thousands and thousands of individual events and episodes, and it is impossible to take them all in. However, many people react or overreact to these events—whether within or beyond their control—as if they were all equally important. They are not. An insignificant slight in the morning need not set off a day-long chain reaction of self-defeating thoughts that can only lead to psychological and immune system stress. Selectively eliminate factors that are merely, if you look at them objectively, little disturbances.

Get enough exercise and sleep. Exercise not only tones the body but raises the levels of endorphins in the bloodstream. These brain chemicals are *naturally* produced mood elevators. Toned stomach and back muscles give support to pelvic organs and strengthen and tone the area. If you do not care for exercise, try a system like yoga, which establishes a contemplative and calming environment as well as an excellent program for toning muscles and gaining flexibility. A third choice is brisk walking, a mild aerobic exercise that can be done at any time, giving it the special benefit of fitting into your schedule.

Fatigue is wearing on the immune system, often creating a secondary stress: overloading on stimulants to stay awake. These are usually coffee, colas, chocolate, sugar in any form, and, for some, drugs like amphetamines. Women with endometriosis have complained of insomnia. This is not uncommon, especially premenstrually. Hormone fluctuations, particularly a sudden surge in estrogen, can trigger a chain of reactions, sometimes causing a disturbance in the brain's "sleep center." Sleep disturbances other than insomnia that are related to pain are increasingly common for sufferers of endometriosis.

Kay Hurlbutt, R.N., M.S.N., prepared a noteworthy clinical paper focused on the self-care aspects of pain management. In her survey, assisted in part by the Endometriosis Association in Milwaukee, Ms. Hurlbutt reported that 100 percent of respondents to her questionnaire said they suffered from pain in various degrees at different days of the month. And it was pain that "interfered in some ways with all aspects of daily life." The most frequently reported disturbance was interference with sleep. Of the respondents, 78 percent reported either difficulty in falling asleep or waking during the night because of pain.

There is a natural approach to relaxing, healthful sleep that is drug-free and, one hopes, pain-free or pain-reduced. The key words to remember are *B complex vitamins* (to offset immune system stress during the day), *calcium* (a natural calmative), *relaxation techniques* (for psychological balance), the brain chemical *serotonin,* and the amino acid *tryptophan.*

Chapter 9 explains further why diet and vitamin-mineral supplements can ease the discomforts associated with menstruation and lessen the pain of endometriosis. For now, concentrate on serotonin and tryptophan, which are thought to be natural mood elevators, produced by the body. Serotonin is considered one of the principle neurotransmitters associated with depression. It has an amino acid precursor, tryptophan, which is crucial to the manufacture of serotonin in the brain.

Tryptophan is found naturally in cow's milk, turkey, tuna and some carbohydrate-high foods like apples. Breast milk, too, is especially high in this amino acid—one reason why infants fall asleep after feeding. Supplying tryptophan to the *adult* body, though, is more than a matter of ingesting any of these foods before bedtime or taking it in concentrated form in capsules.

One theory connects carbohydrate cravings to depletion levels of serotonin. If the level is low enough and the craving urgent enough, the body can get its needed supply expeditiously. It has also been found that tryptophan is best synthesized when it is taken alone or with other carbohydrates; protein, turkey especially, can produce a sense of sleepiness, but studies show that protein will tend to produce counteractive amino acids that will block the passage of tryptophan to the brain.

Does tryptophan really work as a natural mood regulator? In his book *The Brain,* Richard Restak, M.D., describes a number of experiments with volunteers, some of whom took serotonin and some of whom took placebos. Tests were inconclusive. *Yes,* serotonin improved signs of depression in one test, but *no,* there was no overall difference in mood alteration in another. "Relating a subtle disorder of the emotions to disruptions in certain key brain neurotransmitters" is helpful, Dr. Restak reported, but, he added, a decrease of serotonin, for example, can be the result of several causes. "Perhaps," he says, "not enough of the substance is being synthesized, or too much is being broken down. Or perhaps, it isn't being released from its storage vesicles. Or the uptake mechanisms may be overworking." Each of these ideas opens a host of possible explanations as to why *all* volunteers did not uniformly feel better, and why some felt no change whatsoever.

Can tryptophan work for you? Body chemistry is unique and tryptophan is not an absolute mood elevator for everyone. If a low serotonin level signals the onset of depression, then it may be worth your while to increase your intake of tryptophan and see if you are improving on it. The results of Dr. Restak's experiment, in effect, mirror my own observations of tryptophan's effectiveness. Some of my patients respond to tryptophan supplements and others report that they feel no better for having taken them. It is then a matter of experimentation for you, depending on the severity of your menstrual cramps, the degree of sleeplessness, and the extent of mood change.

For the most effective results, take tryptophan forty-five minutes or so before bedtime. Though the tryptophan in milk *can* help you relax, you'd actually require about six or seven glasses of milk to get the same effect as from a standard dosage in supplement tablets. Keep the dosage within reasonable limits. You can safely take two 500-mg capsules of tryptophan midcycle if you suffer from mittelschmerz pain; with the familiar stirrings of PMS symptoms or depression that is harder to cope with, increase the dosage up to twice that, or four capsules a day. Take the first two capsules with a balanced B complex formula pill, whether in tablet or dissolvable brewer's yeast powder. Take the second two with a warm caffeine-free drink like Pero or Postum (which are grain-based beverages).

Linking depression or mood swings to a brain chemical as specific as serotonin has not been proved true in all cases in the way that insulin, for example, is irrevocably connected to blood sugar levels. Brain chemistry is still arcane territory, and experiments continue. Meanwhile, many sufferers of endometriosis, unaware of the natural approach, turn to drugs.

Many sleep disturbances have led women to rely on chemical palliatives, like sleeping pills, tranquilizers, and antidepressants. For a while, Valium was the catch-all pill for PMS and for women who were diagnosed (or undiagnosed) as having endometriosis. Although low-dose tranquilizers may be helpful for chronic sleep disturbances related to pain, I would not recommend them for daily use. Tranquilizers may become addictive for some women and in others may induce the very symptoms they are meant to relieve. Antidepressants—used for treatment of deeper psychological problems—need not be a consideration at all when women follow the vitamin and mineral guidelines and dietary changes suggested in these pages.

If you try the natural approach and you feel you still need medical assistance in falling asleep, your doctor may prescribe Halcion, a mild insomnia tablet; dosage should be one .25-mg or .5-mg tablet. A mild tranquilizer with the palindromic name of Xanax (alprazolam) can be prescribed in .25-mg and .5-mg tablets. I suggest a reasonable dosage of one pill, two (never than three) times a day, but carefully follow your doctor's instructions on dosage. In cases of extreme anxiety, unrelieved by diet, counseling, or Xanax, I would suggest either one of these low-dosage antidepressants *to be taken only occasionally:* Tofranil (imipramine hydrochloride) or Elavil (amitriptyline) in 25-mg tablets to be taken three times a day for a brief period of time.

Let me emphasize that the natural approach will serve as the best mood regulator.

Coping: How Are You Managing Stress?

Your pulse and heartbeat quicken, your blood pressure rises, adrenaline pours into the bloodstream, and body temperature even rises. You suffer bouts of sleeplessness, and your diaphragm muscles tense, causing shortness of breath. What has happened? You are responding physiologically to emotion-arousing stimuli that can short-circuit your productivity, make you susceptible to stress-related disorders such as chronic headaches, eating disorders, depression, stiff neck or backaches, sweating, and ulcers, as well as influence the severity of endometriosis.

You can avoid getting caught in a "nutcracker squeeze." This is a situation in which you feel that the decisions you make about work, coping with health problems, and the ups and downs of your personal life just add greater tension, and do not bring about a resolution that frees you from it. To help you sort out what specific problems apply to you, I have prepared the following quizzes. The answers you provide may give you the information you need to begin making changes that count in conquering your endometriosis.

Answer yes or no to the statements below:

Coping with Endometriosis: What Are Your Attitudes?

1. I don't know why, but I sometimes feel humiliated about having this disease.
2. Sometimes I think that I'm getting so used to having this disease that I cannot imagine being well again.
3. I worry that my endometriosis is really worse than my doctor is telling me.
4. My doctor told me I have endometriosis, but I refuse to believe it can happen to me.
5. I have lied to two doctors about my symptoms. I am afraid to have surgery. If I tell them about all my aches and pains, I know I will hear the worst.
6. When I am told that endometriosis may be a part of my life until menopause, I do my best to tune it out.
7. I don't need any medical attention for my endometriosis. If I ignore it, it will eventually fade away, like a bruise.
8. What really bothers me most about endometriosis is that it is a *chronic* disorder, and no matter what I do, it will always be with me.
9. I don't understand what my doctor tells me about my condition. He says to trust him, so I do.
10. I worry that if I start on some medication for endometriosis, it won't work; then I'll be put on another, and that one won't work either. What if I wind up spending my time and money on worthless treatments? I'll stick with aspirin.
11. I used to be intimidated by my doctor, but I knew that if I

wanted to get rid of endometriosis, I would have to speak up and ask him questions that counted for me.

12. I am always worried about what my doctor will tell me about my condition, but I want to know the truth. I bring along a friend or relative with me to his office to ask all the questions for me.

13. I do not like having this disease, and I refuse to let it run my life.

14. I used to feel sorry for myself about having this disease, but I discovered that self-pity would not make me healthy again.

15. I don't like taking medication, but if it will help me, I will try it for the course of treatment.

16. I used to just talk about how bad endometriosis made me feel. Now I talk about what I can do to feel better.

17. I feel angry that this disease can make me infertile. I have always wanted children and wonder if it is too late for me at this stage of my disease.

18. I get a bit confused about the drugs, the treatments, the possible types of surgery, and the effects of the disease on me. Sometimes it seems as if there are too many options and too many decisions to make.

19. I was surprised to hear that I can actually influence the cure of my endometriosis.

20. I want to do everything I can to fight this disease. To me, nothing is worse than becoming an invalid by withdrawing and surrendering to the pain.

Coping with Work-related Stress: What Matters, What Doesn't?

1. I seem to get all the "junk" work to do from all over the office. My boss says to be flattered by this, since it happens because I'm so efficient.

2. I have a hard time competing for a better job. I tend to diminish my selling points. I tell my boss I want the money, instead of telling him how much I'm doing for the company.

3. I get through the week at a job I dislike more and more each day by planning how to spend my paycheck.

4. I take my job seriously, but my boss doesn't take *me* seriously.

5. I would desperately like a promotion, but I refuse to play politics. Why is business just a game of wits and greed? It sure looks like I won't be asked to play in the game.

6. I got a raise and a promotion, but many people at work still treat me like a secretary. I get hurt and tend to withdraw instead of speaking up.

7. Why do I always wind up working for a demanding dictator who can never be pleased? No matter how hard I work, I am never good enough by his standards.

8. My boss is great at flattering me to get a lot of work out of me; then she takes all the credit for what I've done.

9. I work in a small company that is run like a turn-of-the-century sweatshop. My boss is cheap, he won't answer questions, he keeps changing his mind about what he wants and what my duties are. I go home "wrecked."

10. My boss keeps finding ways to slow me down. I can never seem to get ahead and I'm blamed for the delays.

11. My boss is short-tempered and tends to yell at me. Since I basically like my job, I try to take his outbursts as unemotionally as possible. Instead of yelling back, I respond calmly by explaining *my* side.

12. My boss asks me to do personal errands for him during my lunch hour. If I am busy, I offer to help him find someone else to do them.

13. I explain to my boss or coworkers if I am frustrated or confused about a project, instead of wasting time trying to figure out what is to be done.

14. I used to be everyone's "mother" at work and would spend too much time listening to others' problems. I'd get so behind at the office, I'd have to take my work home. Now I tell office friends when it's not a convenient time for a talk.

15. I work with people who always have excuses for not doing their part. At one time, I would have to beg, nag, threaten, or "joke" the work out of them. Now I call a meeting and tell them when it is due and why it is an urgent matter.

16. I had a hard time taking criticism on the job and denied that anything was wrong with me. I see now that I had a problem *listening* to what should have been done.

17. I keep my desk organized by following a written plan of action each day. It is rewarding to see each job done and crossed off the list.

18. I would like a high-power position at my company. I know I cannot be shy or secretive about my goal and pretend my ambition doesn't exist.

19. Sometimes I get scared by the amount of responsibility I have at the office and do time-wasting "tidying up" to avoid the actual job at hand. I know it's not in my best interest to do this, but that's okay. At least I'm aware of my actions and don't let myself feel bad about them for very long.

20. I have finally learned how to say no graciously, without feeling as if I must go on and on with excuses and apologies to my boss or coworkers.

Coping with Personal Stress: Managing Your Personal Life

1. I tend to be a dreamer, but my dreams look nothing like my life. I wish I knew how to change my life.

2. Somehow, I always wind up taking another person's advice about what to do, even if I don't want to do it. I think that if I ask them for advice, they'll be hurt if I don't take it.

3. People tell me that I never actually tell them what I want or think, but hint around or make suggestions. I don't understand why I need to go into great explanations all the time.

4. I have a feeling that no matter what I do, life for me will remain the same. My mother always says that your future is your past and your present, and that is not what I want.

5. I worry about being a "good" person and whether others think well of me.

6. My husband/lover/parents/children tell me I'm selfish when I do not do as they ask, but do something for myself. I regret it for weeks.

7. I am very dependent on my husband and worry about going out on my own. To me, being single and alone is the worst state a woman can be in.

8. I want children, but I'm afraid to be a mother.

9. When I'm feeling depressed, angry, or lonely, it's easier to turn to chocolate or any sugary food for comfort than express my feelings. No one's really interested, anyway. I'm not one of those women who can run to a gym and work it out that way.

10. I've lost interest in sex and worry that my libido is gone forever.

11. I live in the present and try not to let past problems get in the way of enjoying life. I know that reliving events of the past in my head will not change them for the better.

12. I live in the present, but I look toward a reasonable view of the future that includes realizable goals. I do not hold on to a fatalistic point of view that dooms me in some way to repeat the past, even against my will.

13. I have learned, or I'm working on perfecting, the ability to give

99

myself permission to relax. Sometimes this means I must ask others to wait, but I can take the time I am entitled to and cool down.

14. I no longer have unrealistic expectations about my husband/lover/parents/children. I try to accept them as they are. I know that others can change only when *they* are ready and able to.

15. By being a perfectionist, I tend to place enormous pressures on myself. I am trying to accept my own shortcomings and give up some of the self-defeating thoughts that make me feel inadequate when I'm not.

16. I know I am lovable and no longer feel that I have to do things for others so they will accept me.

17. I know my husband/lover/parents work hard and suffer stress and tension from their jobs, too. When they come home upset, I try not to argue with them and perpetuate the bad feelings, increasing the stress for both of us.

18. I know my mother/sister/grandmother is not directly responsible for my having endometriosis. I do not blame them for any bouts of pain I may suffer from the disease or make *them* feel bad about what none of us could control.

19. If I ever need to go to a pain management clinic, I would want my husband/lover/parent/child to join me in a few sessions. It would make me feel better knowing they understand what I am going through.

20. When I need a supportive person to help me through a situation, I know whom to call. This person is totally on my side and is never undermining.

Statements 1 to 10 in each category indicate a defeated, self-deprecating point of view about oneself and the diminished ability to cope with work-related or personal stress situations. Saying yes to these questions can put you at a disadvantage in fighting endometriosis. In each case, the focus is on a sense of helplessness about your power to change the conditions at work, at home, and with yourself. Remember, these attitudes increase stress on the body, and when stress is increased, endometriosis can tend to worsen.

Any change in your life has to begin by being kind to yourself, maintaining a sense of humor about yourself and others, and giving up the feeling of being life's victim. One way is by not seeing every word or deed in so serious a light and overresponding to too many situations. This is most true for getting along and getting ahead at work.

Business is based on competition, not philanthropy, and success more often has to do with logistics and learning the language of the profession than how hard you work. This is one fact about the business world that is not likely to be changed. What *can* be changed is how you react. If you feel overburdened on the job—enough so that you feel it is having a bad effect on you physically—take an objective look at the situation. If you feel you are being treated unfairly, assert yourself and *speak up in a calm and informative manner.* If you need assistance in understanding what may be the most effective responses to situations that diminish you and your abilities, seek counseling, take a class in assertiveness training, or read books that map out the roads through office politics.

Statements 11 to 20 in each of the three categories indicate how a woman with endometriosis who has a more positive frame of reference about herself deals with an imperfect work world and manages relationships that depend on mutual understanding of each other's lives. Saying yes to these ten statements indicates a stronger sense of self-esteem and self-accepting behavior. These statements express *realistic doubts* and fears about the future, but without a morbid overlay of doom. Having such doubts is normal.

A good attitude helps you feel more relaxed about life and your place in the scheme of things. When you are stress-free, your body's immune system can work more efficiently and effectively in preventing and curing your endometriosis.

Psychologists working with endometriosis patients report that many of them suffer from a *confusion* of feelings about the disease. This confusion can add to the initial stress of dealing with the pain and any diminished ability to take care of responsibilities on a daily basis. The following is a sample of *emotional* responses women have to the disease. On a separate sheet of paper, check off when you feel these responses.

1. I worry that my endometriosis will recur and this makes me upset. *Never/sometimes/often.*
2. I fluctuate between being angry about this disease when it is at its worst and suffering from crying jags. *Never/sometimes/often.*
3. When I have severe menstrual cramps, I suddenly feel a loss of control over my body. *Never/sometimes/often.*
4. I find that when my endometriosis is bad, I get severely depressed, which just makes the pain worse. *Never/sometimes/often.*
5. Friends tell me I should seek help to deal with the pain, but the

thought of going to a therapist adds to my feeling of helplessness. *Never/sometimes/often.*

6. I get very tired and can't concentrate because of the pain, but I continue to do what I can. *Never/sometimes/often.*

7. I have to cancel plans at the last moment because I am not feeling strong enough or interested enough in going out. *Never/sometimes/often.*

8. I think my family tolerates my condition when the pain gets bad, but I secretly fear they see me as a burden. *Never/sometimes/often.*

9. I know it can be hard for my friends and family to talk about how I feel because of endometriosis and for them to sympathize with me. *Never/sometimes/often.*

10. I am trying to sort out my feelings about this disease so I can let my friends and family know how much they mean to me. *Never/sometimes/often.*

If most of your answers indicate a more positive attitude about your condition, you are many steps ahead. If most of your answers reflect a sense of defeat, now is the time to effectively de-stress your life and help yourself get well by:

- confronting the issues
- seeking assistance when you need it
- learning to detach from the past and look ahead with a measure of optimism
- giving yourself permission to ask for what you want and not play the "victim"
- including relaxation exercises in your life
- following your doctor's plan, and
- taking control of your life

I have personally treated a great number of patients whose endometriosis either worsened or recurred during extremely stressful times due to personal or work-related conflicts. On the other hand, the success rate was greater among women with cases of endometriosis who followed my de-stressing program, which includes a change in diet (this will be detailed in chapter 9). We all have a lot more control of our bodies and our destinies than we realize. The advice in these pages should encourage you to believe that you *can* take charge of certain aspects of your life and become a partner in your health care.

CHAPTER 8

Tuning in to Alternate Therapies

ALTERNATE therapies offer many possible avenues for alleviating the many problems associated with endometriosis. Uppermost among the benefits of these therapies, such as acupuncture, herbal preparations, yoga and other relaxation techniques, may be temporary relief from chronic pain. These medically unorthodox therapies appeal to those women with endometriosis who do not like taking prescription drugs or for those who like to supplement medications with pain-control techniques.

In the last fifteen years or so, there has been greater interest in investigating pain control through behavior modification, self-hypnosis, biofeedback, imaging, and stress management techniques. For the endometriosis sufferer, especially the woman who has severe and *chronic* pain, such a program can guide her toward feeling more in charge of her body and her life. A good pain-control program will address the psychological as well as physiological realities of the disease. A number of pain clinics across the country are affiliated with medical centers, such as the Pain Management Center at UCLA in California, which operates an outpatient Pelvic Pain Program. Other clinics may be privately run. Finding a pain-control program is a matter of asking your doctor or inquiring at a large hospital or medical association.

A good measure of satisfaction comes from having some success with these alternate techniques, since many of them depend on your *commitment* to them in time, energy, and a sense of purpose. Unlike conventional medical therapies, they can be something of a challenge in this regard, but they are fascinating nonetheless. When you learn how to control pain without painkilling drugs, you will understand more about who you are, while having as well the adventure of mastering a new discipline, such as behavior modification, meditation, or yoga.

Many of what are now considered alternate therapies were once the only source of practical medical treatments. They coexist now with supersophisticated surgical techniques (such as laser) and the nearly perfected drugs for treating endometriosis (such as the gonadotropin-releasing hormones, or GnRH, discussed in chapter 10). They remain popular, if not without an aspect of controversy attached to whether or not they work. Let's begin with a sampling of historical modes of treatment.

A Brief Look at Menstrual Cramp Remedies

Lydia Pinkham brought a measure of respectability to over-the-counter menstrual remedies in the 1920s with a tonic designed to help sufferers of monthly ills. Although the tonic was often a staple of medicine chests, like iodine and aspirin, there is some doubt as to whether it was of any real medicinal value, other than providing a psychological boost. This formula preceded the more effective up-to-date menstrual cramp remedies, like ibuprofen.

Before such modern prostaglandin inhibitors were developed, it was not unusual to hear of women who became addicted to laudanum—a tincture of opium—to relieve their pain. Others tried nonmedical treatments like hot sweat baths with massage, hoping to perspire out the disease. The rubdown, or "salt glow," following the bath was concentrated in the abdominal area to stimulate blood flow to the area. "Galvanism," a less fearsome cousin of shock treatment, applied electrical current to the area to reduce pain. Along with the staple family recipes for healing that were handed down generation to generation, liniments, douches, decoctions, poultices, and brews were available from doctors, mail-order catalogs, pharmacies, and quacks.

Modern pharmacology can manufacture drugs from synthetics, plants, minerals, whatever, but turn-of-the-century cures relied on plants. Although few women nowadays partake of hemlock tea (made from the leaves and inner bark) to "tone the uterus," there is a renewed and growing interest among women with endometriosis in drug-free therapies that are as young as TENS (transcutaneous electrical nerve stimulation, a form of biofeedback and stress control) and as old as acupuncture. Some of these therapies require the ministrations of experts on an individual basis; others, like dietary changes and stress management, can be, in general, incorporated into the daily lives of most sufferers of the disease.

Are these therapies effective? Let's examine them, starting with the 5,000-year-old practice of acupuncture.

TREATING ENDOMETRIOSIS WITH ACUPUNCTURE

With its basis in Taoist philosophy, acupuncture first struck Western observers as little more than Chinese folklore or "barefoot medicine." A vast majority of American physicians were dubious about the scientific credibility of this ancient medical system, equating it with superstitious kitchen cures, like chicken soup for colds and flu or pickle juice for removing warts.

Few people heard of acupuncture until *New York Times* columnist James Reston was stricken with appendicitis upon his arrival in Peking about sixteen years ago. His appendix was removed under conventional anesthesia, but the surprise was that Reston agreed to postoperative acupuncture treatment to relieve his abdominal pain. He reported that within an hour and thereafter, he was free of any abdominal pressure or distention. Subsequently, teams of American doctors toured Chinese medical centers to observe the alleged range of acupuncture's capabilities, beyond that of inducing anesthesia. What they found, among other things, was that acupuncture treatments were shown to combat infectious diseases, reputedly by raising the level of bacteria-fighting white blood cells.

How does acupuncture work? In China this needle therapy developed in conjunction with the accompanying practice of moxibustion, or the burning of the herb mugwort, at or near the appropriate points on the patient's body. According to Chinese theory, disease is an imbalance of yin (female) and yang (male) forces disrupting an orderly flow of Ch'i, or energy. Bodily organs as well as behavior, temperature, and other functions are assigned yin or yang attributes. Even the ingestion of food is based on this principle of opposites: there is yin (such as fruit) or yang (such as red meat) as well as foods that are balanced (like brown rice and other grains). Chinese physicians believe that all forces—universal or earthly—influence human organic functions and fluctuations, which will be different for each of us.

Acupuncturists take as truth that energy flows from organ to organ through channels, or meridians, beneath the skin. There are twelve such meridians running on either side of the body, one along the center front and one in back. There are up to eight hundred points spaced systematically along these meridians that acupuncturists must learn to pierce with needles, thereby correcting imbalances in the corresponding organs. Once needles are in place, they may be twirled or not, depending on the complex law governing the relationship between the type of needling and the organs.

The bafflement for many Westerners is that the needles need not be placed anywhere near where the trouble is. For example, acupuncture needles stuck in a specifically designated point on the hand can reduce abdominal cramps, while a needle placed in a governed point around the knee can help kidney function. How could this happen? No one actually knows. In fact, no one knows why acupuncture works at all. Naturally, theories abound to explain it. Dr. Ronald Hoffman, M.D., medical director of the Whole Life Medical Center and a general practitioner in New York City who practices holistic or alternate medicine, including acupuncture, told me: "I think acupuncture is extremely helpful in the treatment of endometriosis, although we don't know exactly what's happening. In Chinese medicine, there is no actual formal diagnosis of endometriosis. But with menstrual problems, such as dysmenorrhea, or painful menstruation, it was considered pelvic congestion or *stagnated* energy. The acupuncture treatment, then, was designed to unblock the channel and release that stagnation."

Should you try acupuncture?

Many patients dislike taking medication, or they find that it is no longer working for them. Others suffer from undesirable side effects. Acupuncture is a relatively benign therapy that may help in some cases for pain management. A study done by Dr. Joseph M. Helms, a family practitioner in Berkeley, California, demonstrated how this ancient treatment may be effective for sufferers of dysmenorrhea.

Dr. Helms set up an experiment in which he divided forty-three women into four groups. One group got *real* acupuncture treatment at appropriate acupuncture points (specific points on the feet, knees, forearms, and lower abdomen). A second group was given *false* acupuncture, that is, at random points on their bodies. A third group was followed without medical attention or acupuncture, and the fourth group just "visited" the project doctor once a month. All of these women were regularly taking medication to control their monthly pain. (Remember, cramps are caused by high prostaglandin levels prompting the uterus to contract. Antidotes for cramps are prostaglandin inhibitors.)

Dr. Helms's study was undertaken for a period of twelve months before tabulating his results: 90.9 percent of those treated with *real* acupuncture (ten out of eleven subjects) showed improvement; four out of eleven given false acupuncture said they felt improved. The *real* acupuncture group reported a decrease in cramping, pain, nausea, headache and backache, and premenstrual symptoms of fluid retention and breast tenderness, and they improved immediately. From his firsthand analysis, Dr. Helms theorizes that acupuncture may work for any number of reasons: the concentration of prostaglandins in the endometrium is altered either *directly* by the stimulation of the acupuncture treatment or "*indirectly* via the concentration of estrogen or progesterone." Again, he reported, it may be some other "neural mechanism triggered by the acupuncture treatments."

Part of such a positive result of acupuncture treatment, Dr. Helms feels, is a "bias of self-selection." This means that it is possible that patients *willing to accept* acupuncture as a valid medical treatment would be more willing to participate in such a study, while those who were against acupuncture were underrepresented.

Nevertheless, the study had an interesting resolution, since most women in these groups wanted to stop taking medication and handle the treatment of pain in some other way. Dr. Hoffman feels that acupuncture can help in certain cases, but that women with endometriosis in an advanced state may get little pain relief.

Acupuncture has mystique, but it's not a miracle cure.

HERBAL REMEDIES: BEYOND CHAMOMILE TEA

Herbs are not simple spices and should be treated with exceptional wisdom and respect. Medicinal herbal cures and treatments are as old as the first amateur botanist who most likely discovered the effects of plants quite by accident. A respectable percentage of modern drugs are made from plants, or were made from plants, before they were artificially reproduced. Penicillin and belladonna are two such drugs; Valium, the tranquilizer, may have had its roots in valerian, an herb known for its identical effect.

How safe, then, are herbs for the woman with endometriosis?

Abigail Rist, a registered nurse and registered acupuncturist with a specialty of herbalism, who has worked with midwives and treated many women with menstrual disorders, believes that sufferers of endometriosis may gain some benefits from a number of herbal remedies. She follows the Chinese school of thought, viewing disease as imbalances of female (yin) and male (yang) energies, heat and cold, expansion and contraction. The herbal teas or tinctures she recommends are based on these evaluations.

Since this system of medicine does not specify the disease precisely, "endometriosis is diagnosed and treated by its more irritating symptoms," Ms. Rist told me. "In this sense, endometriosis is a tightening and overcooling of what is called 'the lower burner,' or urogenital area. For this area, we prepare an herbal remedy to replenish heat (or yang) and reestablish a balance. In another example, it's as if you have a fever or sore throat, accompanied by thirst. The remedy prescribed will bring down body heat, soothe the rawness of the throat, and help quench thirst. Dandelion tea, for example, induces these qualities. The same will be done for endometriosis."

Using this reasoning, the overcooling effects of endometriosis would need to be treated or counteracted with warmth. The herbs used would tonify the blood, stimulate and warm the organs. "In traditional Chinese medicine," Ms. Rist continued, "doctors attribute the function and regulation of some aspects of the blood to the liver and spleen. If a woman has dark clots during menstruation, it is attributed to an imbalance of the liver. If a woman has lighter red blood but profuse bleeding, this would be related to an imbalance of the spleen. The herbs prescribed would be 'tissue specific,' that is, herbs with some affinity to each organ which can, if possible, influence and regulate its function."

There are teas and tinctures that Ms. Rist recommends. The *white peony* has specific liver action, so it will actually decrease abdominal tightness and pain. The peony, which may be either dry-roasted or cured, depending on what the herbalist decides for each case, is often one of four other herbs blended in a concoction and prepared to be taken as tea. "Its nature is to be cooling," says Ms. Rist, "so when it enters the spleen and liver channels, it can tonify the blood. The herbs can also help stop pain by relaxing the tendons and tissues."

Another popularly used herb is *dong quai,* considered a "female" root plant, the way that ginseng is assigned male properties. Dong quai is found in many "female trouble" herb blends that are commercially made and distributed to health food stores. It is a cured root that, says Ms. Rist, "is thought to help establish an endocrine balance, increasing tissue sensitivity to estrogen and helps with ending menstrual cramps and pelvic congestion."

Another tea suggested by this herbalist is *raspberry* tea, handed down as a remedy from grandmother's time to its use by present-day midwives. It is reputed to help relax muscles and dilate the cervix. Other teas that are toning or can help reduce inflammation or relieve pain are *rosemary* tea, *licorice* tea, *chamomile,* and *witch hazel* tea.

HOMEOPATHY: WHEN LIKE CURES LIKE

A medical system all its own, homeopathy treats disease by administration of a minute dose of a remedy that would in a healthy person produce symptoms of the disease being treated. Although homeopaths do not believe in surgery and avoid prescribing prescription drugs, they are trained medical doctors who have also trained in herbalism and nutrition. ("Homeopathy" is practiced, in one way, within the traditional medical establishment. Vaccines against diseases like polio, measles, smallpox, and other contagious and potentially life-threatening diseases are actually comprised of minute qualities of active viruses.) Homeopathically, the body reacts by stimulating the immune system to fight the illness through self-healing. Homeopathic doctors give diluted doses of substances to stimulate the immune system, although vaccines are given to people when they are well, not ill with symptoms of the disease.

Homeopathy, then, uses the familiar technique of "like cures like"; that is, the cure is found within the system of the disorder. One remedy that homeopaths work with in some cases of endometriosis is a distillation of *healthy* human placenta. The placenta is boiled down, then dried and ground to powder form. It is given with other herbs to restore vital essence of the basic life force in the body. It is often given to women who suffer from infertility, excessive menstruation, or lack of menstruation. A homeopathic diagnosis would be necessary to determine the right quantity of placenta for you, or determine if it was right for you at all. In my opinion, homeopathy might work for some women, but would not be right for others. Each case must be viewed individually.

YOGA: A WAY TO RELAXATION

One first associates this ancient Indian discipline with its most famous symbol—the lotus position, a sitting posture with legs folded in a pretzel shape. Yoga is far more than just a series of such very specific postures. It is also, like acupuncture, based on a philosophical system that encompasses cosmic ideologies, theories about life forces and one's control over them, and healing. Yoga, for one, teaches its practitioners to concentrate on deep and rhythmic breathing, which is instrumental for inducing relaxation and an overall sense of well-being. This concentration on taking in *prana,* or the purported vital force that is assimilated into the body through breath control, serves to quiet the mind by diminishing awareness of the external environment. Those who are very practiced at the breathing art, a Yogi or any devotee of the discipline, can learn to drastically slow down their breathing rate as well as alter consciousness to the point of a trance state. For most of us, yoga breathing techniques offer a means to a pleasant sense of tranquillity.

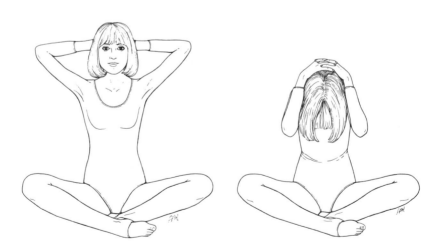

Breathing technique is an essential part of doing yoga exercises, too. These *asanas,* or postures, are designed to strengthen the back, tone muscles, increase flexibility, stimulate nerves and glands, change the direction of blood flow, help in the elimination of waste products, and oxygenate the body through slow breathing. These exercises do not "go for the burn," in the way that energetic calisthenics and aerobics can. Rather, nearly all the postures are static, held for a period of time while breathing rhythmically, and are usually not done in sets of repetitions.

The following two simple yoga exercises can relax and gently stretch the back and pelvic muscles, especially aiding in the relief of menstrual cramps. They are best done along with slow, rhythmic breathing, so do *not* hold your breath as you ease into the postures.

To begin, sit on a low-pile rug or towel; wear an exercise leotard or loose-fitting clothes. Keeping your back straight, cross your legs and clasp your hands behind your head, as shown in the illustration below. Point your elbows out, keep shoulders relaxed and *down* (not hunched), and keep your chest raised (do not collapse in). Breathe in

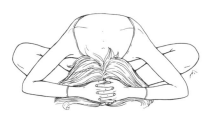 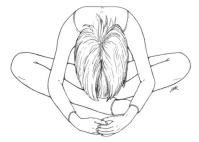

slowly for two counts, then pull in your stomach and begin to round your back slightly. Breathe out, dropping your chin to your chest. Your elbows will be drawn together. Now breathe in again for two counts and return to the starting straight-back posture. Repeat four more times to relax.

As you begin the sixth repeat, breathe in and continue rounding down, bringing your forehead as close to the floor as you can, as shown below. Keep your elbows out to the side. Do not strain, bounce, or pull your head down with your clasped hands. Keep your stomach tucked in. Breathe slowly and rhythmically.

Extend your arms in front of you, as shown in the fourth illustration. Breathe slowly for the count of five, then roll up to the original sitting pose. Repeat the entire set three times.

For the next exercise, lie flat on your back. Bend both knees, lightly clasping each knee, as shown below. Relax your feet, take a breath, and then let it out slowly. Lightly pull your knees close to your chest (see illustration). Breathe in and out slowly for a count of five, then release

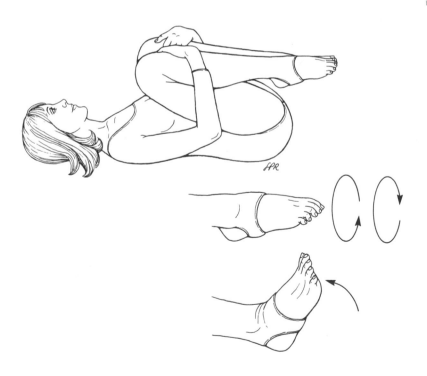

knees to starting position. Now point your toes and rotate your feet from the ankle, circling outwardly five times. Now flex your foot five times, as shown. Repeat the exercise, circling your feet inwardly five times and flexing your feet five times. This exercise helps increase circulation and relieves menstrual cramps, so you may repeat it fully five times. Then stretch out and breathe quietly for a few minutes. If your cramps are severe, do another set.

Yoga is best learned at first with a teacher's guidance, rather than through a book. Yoga looks easy and sounds simple, but you will get more out of it with the help of an expert. He or she can give you tips about body alignment and show you how to get in and out of the postures properly and safely. Yoga classes are frequently offered at Y's, through adult education programs, and at dance studios, and are taught by individuals who have studied the system and have mastered it. There is also yoga instruction on videotape for home use, including one led by Raquel Welch.

MEDITATION FOR STRESS CONTROL

Meditation was brought to the Western world from India by the Maharishi Mahesh Yogi, the guru, or spiritual leader, who taught a mind-control technique known as TM, or transcendental meditation. Unlike yoga and acupuncture, which are rooted in more religious connected systems and philosophies, meditation is considered a *natural approach* to reducing stress, inducing therapeutic healing, and expanding awareness. TM's relaxation techniques help alter brain waves, control heart rate, stimulate circulation, decrease muscle tension, and lower the levels of blood lactate levels. A natural byproduct of inefficient cell metabolism, lactate levels in excess have been linked to chronic overproduction of adrenaline, anxiety attacks, and high-stress living. Researchers investigating TM's beneficial qualities reported cases that included reduction of high blood pressure, improvement of asthmatic conditions and gastrointestinal problems, fewer sleep disturbances, and even improvement in learning ability and general mental health.

This is quite a menu of benefits. How does TM work to effect such a range of changes? To meditate, one sits with eyes closed, feet flat on the floor, most preferably in a silent room, although many practitioners can meditate in public places, including planes, waiting rooms, and doctor's offices. To help bring about the paradoxical state of deep rest with increased wakefulness, you must shift your awareness inward and tune out the environment. This sensation has been likened to that near suspension of complete consciousness before falling asleep. To aid in concentration, some people picture an imaginary spot on their foreheads and focus on that; others may disengage from the outside world by either silently or vocally repeating a word that has been especially selected for them by a TM instructor. This sound "syllable," such as the widely used "om," is called a *mantra*.

TM is a good relaxation technique, thought best practiced twice a day for about fifteen minutes each time. It may help the woman with endometriosis and sufferers of premenstrual syndrome, too.

If you are being treated by a doctor for endometriosis, it is always advisable to let him know about any alternate choices you want to make in your health care. This helps him to better monitor your condition and facilitate healing.

The Endometriosis Diet
That Helps Healing

What you eat can change the course of endometriosis enough to make a difference in your life.

The effect of diet on the body is no longer just an issue of sustenance for survival. It is also a matter of health, and even longer life. We know, fairly conclusively, that high cholesterol levels affect heart function, high-fat diets may be connected to bowel and breast cancer, and that salt irrevocably influences blood pressure. Each year, there is more evidence of how certain foods and vitamins have the ability to fuel our immune systems, while other nutrients, or nonnutrients such as caffeine, can cause us problems.

Women with endometriosis, especially those who are enduring chronic pain, may not be eating correctly. This could be more from a lack of appetite or lack of energy than from a lack of knowledge as to what is best to eat. This may also be true of women with mild endometriosis. Nutrition affects recovery rates from disease, and the low-fat, low-salt, low-sugar diet and vitamin plan that I have designed for endometriosis sufferers can make a difference.

Before we get to the actual diet plan, you should know why you will be taking minerals, vitamins, and selected nutritional supplements. These dietary changes will most benefit any woman with endometriosis. Let's break it down to specifics.

THE GOOD OILS

Although no conclusive data exists yet, many doctors and nutritionists feel they are going in the right direction by recommending limited intake of arachidonic acid and supplements of gamma-linolenic acid, or GLA, to women with endometriosis.

Arachidonic acid is an essential fatty acid that is linked to inflammatory conditions, as is the case with endometriosis. What does this mean to you? Inflammation is often mediated by prostaglandins. Knowing this, many doctors are suggesting to patients that they eliminate foods containing this acid, which is found in dietary sources of saturated fat, such as butter, animal and organ meats, and lard. It is also possible to alter the balance of arachidonic acid by taking another oil to counteract its effect. This is where linolenic acid comes in.

Found in sources as diverse as mother's milk and cold-pressed safflower oil, gamma-linolenic acid, or GLA, is one of the body's more essential fatty acids. It is most important for the woman with endometriosis, both as a possible pain inhibitor and as an immune system strengthener.

GLA is made in the body from a conversion of vitamin F, or linolenic acid, which is the basis of prostaglandins. Prostaglandins E2 and F2 Alpha have been linked to uterine contractions producing menstrual cramps, while GLA, called prostaglandin E1, may offset some of the worse symptoms of the opposing prostaglandins. In a number of studies, it was also found to oppose the constriction of blood vessels, prevent blood clots, and prevent cholesterol buildup in the arteries. It has also been tried experimentally to help alcoholics over their addiction and to reduce some of the irritation of eczema.

Suggestions for daily intake: Take one to two tablespoons of safflower, walnut, or *nutritional* linseed oil (*not* the commercial variety used for varnishes) a day, preferably on a fresh tossed salad, flavored with herbs. Follow with a tablet of vitamin E to help absorption. GLA is also available as evening primrose oil—either the essence of oil or in 500-mg tablets. You should be aware that this oil is very costly (approximately thirty dollars for 180 tablets) and may not be much more effective than a daily salad with the above-mentioned oils.

MINERALS

While about 96 percent of the body is water, protein, and fats, the remaining 4 percent is accounted for by minerals. When we think of minerals, the first one that comes to mind is calcium. Others include magnesium, phosphorus, zinc, iodine, potassium, and sodium. Hard skeletal structure is composed primarily of minerals, but we could not survive or reproduce without adequate and balanced amounts of the minerals that form the nuclei of soft tissues such as muscle and nerve cells.

Minerals are responsible for regulating a few crucial functions, such as nerve responses, and for maintaining the acid–base equilibrium that helps in the absorption of minerals and contraction of muscles.

Calcium

While calcium is the most abundant mineral in the body, it is most likely to be deficient in diets. Only 1 percent of body calcium is found in the blood, other fluids, and soft tissues. Its presence in proper proportion with sodium, potassium, and magnesium is necessary for contraction of muscle fibers and maintenance of heartbeat rhythm. Calcium is also considered a muscle relaxant and soporific for the nerves.

Calcium levels in menstruating women tend to drop about ten to fourteen days before onset of a period. Unless there is an increase in calcium intake at this time, there could be a temporary deficiency that induces headaches, muscle cramps, depression or mood swings, bloating, and pelvic pain. Therefore, a woman with endometriosis will particularly want to monitor her calcium intake.

Calcium absorption is tricky, since this function is related to the intake of magnesium and vitamin D and takes place only in the small intestine. Vitamin D increases optimum absorption of this mineral; however, a number of dietary factors can interfere with absorption, including the presence of phytic and oxalic acids. A woman on a high-fat diet or with a poor ability to digest fat, or someone on a very high fiber diet, can inadvertently set up circumstances that will interfere with calcium absorption. This is why: oxalic acid, an organic acid occurring naturally in such foods as spinach, beet greens, cocoa, and rhubarb, combines with calcium to form an insoluble salt that renders the calcium unavailable to the body. Chocolate milk, for example, may be delicious, but the cocoa can be calcium depleting; and spinach, while a wonderful source of calcium, contains within its own chemistry enough oxalic acid to lessen its dietary calcium! Phytic acid is found in the bran layer of grains and also combines with calcium to make it unavailable. Whole-grain cereals, then, should *not* be consumed with high-calcium foods like milk.

The parathyroid hormone maintains a constant blood calcium concentration. When blood calcium is reduced, the mineral can be mobilized from bone, and when the blood level is increased, calcium is excreted by the kidneys. Many women who are worried about osteoporosis, one result of skeletal calcium deficiency, are taking calcium supplements. *Can you take too much calcium?* Oversupplies of unabsorbed calcium may be excreted in urine and stools. If you have a kidney disorder or any other condition that will demand attentiveness to calcium intake, check with your doctor. It is wise to do this, in fact, before taking *any* mineral supplements to relieve some symptoms of endometriosis.

The best food sources of calcium have typically been milk and dairy products, followed by green leafy vegetables and some types of fish. An excellent low-calorie, high-calcium drink without a trace of caffeine is *bancha tea,* otherwise known as green twig tea or kukicha tea. A 3–4-ounce serving of this tea contains more than 700 mg of calcium—or two and one-half times the calcium of the same quantity of whole milk. Bancha is brewed by steeping a few teaspoons of the delicate, cut-up twigs in boiling water for a few minutes. It has a light tea favor, contains virtually no calories, and is a nutritious tonic drink. You can buy bancha tea at a health food store and enjoy a cup or two a day.

Dosage: For severe uterine cramping and nervous irritability, you may do better with calcium supplements to get maximum dosage. If you prefer calcium supplements, my choices among the many calcium compounds are calcium gluconate and bonemeal tablets. Drink at least one cup of hot or cold unsweetened brancha tea.

Calcium gluconate: For cramps take two 500-mg tablets twice daily; more than four tablets (or 2,000 mg) is not necessarily better, and do not exceed six tablets (3,000 mg) a day. Take calcium with 350 mg of magnesium, 1,000 units of vitamin D, and 100 mg of phosphorus.

Bonemeal: Bonemeal compounds often come in already balanced formulas. Check the labels to be sure it contains vitamin D, phosphorus, and magnesium, or add supplements as you need them. Begin taking two or three bonemeal tablets per day about ten days before your menstrual period, continuing them through your cycle.

Best selection of foods with calcium: Dairy foods are prime sources of calcium, but since their fat content may be implicated in exacerbating symptoms of endometriosis, the wiser course is to *reduce* intake for ten days a month. Begin lowering the amount of these products a week before your menstrual period is due and during the cycle. You may want to have soy products one day and alternate these with a limited amount of dairy products the next. Other than milk, cheese, and yogurt, excellent sources are bancha tea, canned salmon (with bones), clams, broccoli, turnips, greens, and kale.

Phosphorus

Second in rank after calcium in the amount present in the body, phosphorus has been found to have more functions than any other mineral. About 80 percent of it will combine with calcium to strengthen bone structure, and the remainder nourishes soft tissues and bodily fluids. Among its important functions is to help metabolize fats and carbohydrates and fuel muscle energy metabolism. Unfortunately, many high-phosphorus foods are anathema for the endometriosis sufferer, since they tend to be high in fat and cholesterol. These include egg yolk, red meat, and whole-milk cheeses. Other foods are better bets, such as lean turkey breast and whole-grain cereals. Fruit, which you want to limit during the menstrual cycle and the ten days preceding it, is low in phosphorus, as are most vegetables. (Fruits contain bioflavinoids, which can mimic the effect of estrogen in the body.) If you have enough calcium and protein in your diet, you should be getting enough phosphorus.

Magnesium

There is 100 to 200 times as much calcium as magnesium in bones, but muscles contain about 3 times as much magnesium as calcium. Magnesium deficiency has been found in alcoholics and in people suffering from kidney disorders and may be responsible, in part, for endometriotic discomfort and PMS. The endometriotic woman experiencing a magnesium deficiency might have bouts of insomnia, nervousness, rapid heartbeat, muscle cramping, and abdominal menstrual cramping. One of magnesium's functions is to regulate body temperature, and large quantities of this mineral can be lost through perspiration—whether because of overheated rooms, hot weather, or exercising.

Dosage: Magnesium and calcium must be present in the proper proportion of 2:1—that is, the body needs twice the dosage of calcium as magnesium. If magnesium intake is increased, it should be kept to *half* the calcium intake. To help ease cramping, take one 500-mg tablet of calcium gluconate along with 250 mg of magnesium.

Best selection of foods with magnesium: soybeans, brussels sprouts, wheat germ, brewer's yeast, peanuts, leafy vegetables, brown rice.

Zinc

Zinc is present in all human tissue and known to be an essential mineral for successful enzyme activity in the body. Zinc is also responsible for helping our cells reproduce. Without zinc, RNA and DNA, which are critical components of each body cell, will not develop correctly. Zinc deficiency affects the immune system and our resistance to infection, impeding the body's healing process by weakening white blood cells. Wounds, for example, cannot heal properly without zinc. Studies link a deficiency of this mineral to some cases of infertility in both women *and* men. In fact, the highest concentration of zinc in the body is found in the prostate gland. During the premenstrual and menstrual cycle, a zinc deficiency can induce headaches, depression, and irritability.

Dosage: Since zinc can help the woman with endometriosis negotiate the world with a greater sense of well-being and better spirits under stressful times, I'd recommend a 50-mg tablet per day, increased to (but not to exceed) 100 mg for at least ten days before the menstrual cycle. Take zinc with calcium and magnesium. Do not take iron pills at the same time, since these minerals tend to counteract each other's absorption into the bloodstream.

Best selection of foods with zinc: Zinc is most notably found in shellfish, especially oysters, and in organ meats like liver, as well as in nuts and whole-grain cereals.

Potassium

Red blood cells and muscle tissue are rich with potassium. Together with calcium and magnesium, potassium regulates the contraction of muscles, regular heartbeat and the conduction of nerve impulses, and the maintenance of fluid balance. Potassium, like sodium, is considered an electrolyte—that is, a dissolved salt or alkali that plays a crucial role in maintaining fluid balance and stabilizing brain chemistry. Potassium is the chief mineral in the cells. With sodium, it controls the amount of fluid retention. It helps offset the effects of sodium in individuals with high blood pressure. Potassium can be lost if you suffer from diarrhea during an especially trying bout of endometriosis. One bonus of potassium is that it tends to be well distributed in both animal and plant foods, so a well-balanced diet should provide enough during normal times. During stressful attacks of the "career woman's disease," though, you may experience a change in balance of these minerals.

Bloating (or edema), weakness, and fatigue may occur because of potassium deficiency, and a restoration of the sodium-potassium balance can be beneficial.

Dosage: Potassium is available in liquid or tablet form. Potassium gluconate tablets contain 5 milliequivalents (mEq) of potassium gluconate. My recommended dose is two tablets four times daily, after meals and at bedtime. This will supply 40 mEq of potassium, which is the minimum daily requirement. The liquid dosage of two tablespoons daily provides approximately 20 mEq of potassium gluconate per tablespoon.

If you are suffering from kidney or cardiovascular disorders, be advised that a high potassium level can result in an irregular heartbeat or even death from heart failure. Always consult your doctor before embarking on this or any vitamin-mineral program. Potassium also has been known to be a stomach irritant. Both the pills and the liquid, now available in a syrup base that offsets gastrointestinal upset, should be taken with meals.

Best selection of foods with potassium: Excellent sources of potassium include bananas, apricots, oranges, dried fruits, peanuts, potatoes, dark green leafy vegetables, and chicken.

Iron

Iron can be the most important mineral during a woman's reproductive years. Iron is essential to the function of red blood cells and hemoglobin, the vehicle that carries oxygen in your blood. The life cycle of red blood cells is about one hundred days. All women, especially those leading active lives, need an adequate supply of iron. Women naturally have 600,000 fewer red blood cells per milliliter than men. Women store less iron, too: comparatively, women store 250 mg of iron while the average man stores 830 mg. Women on the average lose about 30 mg of iron per menstrual period, but a woman with endometriosis who is also suffering from heavy bleeding, clots, breakthrough bleeding, sweating, and stress adds to her risk of iron deficiency or some degree of anemia. Symptoms of iron deficiency are weakness, extreme physical fatigue, and mental exhaustion.

Dosage: The body does not absorb all the iron you take in. In fact, it is estimated that only about 10 percent of this mineral is absorbed! You can see how not taking an adequate amount might cause serious problems. If heavy bleeding is symptomatic of your case of endometriosis, begin with iron supplements taken in ferrous gluconate tablets. Health food shops and drugstores will also offer a less easily absorbed form of iron as ferrous sulfate. Natural iron can be found in preparations like yeast or desiccated liver in tablet or powder form, allowing you to build up to a greater dosage over a greater length of time. The recommended daily allowance for adult women of reproductive years is 18 mg—a ludicrously low nutritional "requirement" under the circumstances. Rather, I would recommend taking 40–50 mg a day *during* menstruation. If you suffer from breakthrough bleeding too, take 20–25 mg during that time. Divide the dosage into two portions and take it with your two largest meals. To ensure better absorption of iron, take 500 to 1,000 mg of vitamin C equally divided between two doses per day, or take the iron with a vegetable or fruit rich in vitamin C. (See the vitamin and mineral chart, pages 134–135.)

If you don't feel stronger after a month of iron supplements, check with your doctor to see if you might be suffering from anemia due to a vitamin B_{12} deficiency or malabsorption of iron. Do not simply increase your dosage of iron. This is one supplemental nutrient that should *not* be taken in megadoses—it will cause greater harm than good. Side effects of excessive iron intake can range from stomach cramps, fainting, and diarrhea to damage to the kidneys, liver, and heart.

Best selection of foods with iron: When cooked, organ meats like beef liver and kidneys can be savory, but while they are very high in iron content they also are high in cholesterol and calories. Another iron-rich food, egg yolk, bears a similar curse. If you are watching fat intake and calories, limit these foods and concentrate on other sources of dietary iron such as whole grains, dried apricots, potatoes, and, as an old-fashioned treat, a tablespoon of blackstrap molasses.

Sodium

Along with sugar and fat, American diets are too liberal with salt, or sodium chloride. We would perish without some salt, since it functions to balance water between our cells and helps maintain blood pressure. Simply, salt binds water. If sodium intake is restricted, our kidneys will conserve body sodium by excreting very little of it. The amount of sodium that is excreted by the kidneys is controlled by the adrenal cortical hormone. If sodium levels are too high, extra fluid will build up in the heart and blood vessels, forcing the heart to work harder and increasing blood pressure. Along with this, a premenstrual increase of blood estrogen promotes sodium retention, which explains the feeling of being bloated or waterlogged at this time of the menstrual cycle. Fluid retention also contributes to a sense of irritability. If bloating is extreme, a woman may be advised by her doctor to take a diuretic during her menstrual period to relieve symptoms.

Dosage: Table salt is the most accessible form of sodium, although it is considered more a condiment or spice than a mineral. Many of us overindulge in salt, consuming 2–3 teaspoons of it a day (4–5 grams) or more while we only require about half that for normal functioning. You'll be on the safe side if you limit salt consumption to under a teaspoon a day—the equivalent of about 2,000 mg—and half a teaspoon premenstrually and during the menstrual cycle.

A selection of foods to avoid with high sodium content: Foods high in salt content include those that are cured and pickled (bacon, ham, sausage, corned beef, pickles, sauerkraut) and carbonated beverages (sodas, including plain seltzer unless the bottle is otherwise marked low—or no—sodium). Canned vegetables, canned soups, and canned vegetable juices are prepared at manufacturing plants where they are salted by an overly generous hand. Some dairy products like ice cream, cottage cheese, cheddar, Brie, and many other soft or hard cheeses supply in a portion enough salt to make a difference. You'll also discover sodium in tablets for indigestion, some laxatives, and other over-the-counter medications. Women with endometriosis are advised to avoid these foods and preparations at least a week before and during their menstrual cycles.

Finally, before buying any packaged food or frozen meals, do some sleuthing and check the label for sodium content. Salt is 40 percent sodium, and it is this element that should concern you when you see it listed as an ingredient. Salt may be "hidden" in sodium compounds used as preservatives (such as sodium diacetate) or as a flavoring or flavor enhancer (monosodium glutamate). If the label instructs you that the sodium content for a serving of canned tomato soup is 1,000 mg, be aware that you have just had half your daily dose. Be alert to how you will consume salt for the remainder of the day to keep your intake to a minimum.

Selenium

Selenium, like iron, zinc, iodine, and fluorine, is a trace mineral, or micromineral, and is not needed in greater quantities for health. While microminerals are essential to health in trace amounts, they exist in the body in minute quantities. In fact, *all* trace minerals weighed together would add up to only about .01 percent of your total body weight. Few of us knew of selenium's role in immune system function until about five years ago when Durk Pearson and Sandy Shaw popularized their findings about this little-known mineral in their book *Life Extension,* which concentrated on antiaging processes through nutritional supplement dosing and megadosing. Among the dozen or so properties they described for this mineral was that in various formulas, selenium could not only slow down the aging process but also might prevent breast cancer, help alcoholics fight their addiction, lessen stiffness and pain for arthritis victims, and, most important, strengthen the immune system.

Selenium is an antioxidant, as are the vitamins C and E. This means that selenium is important in preventing complications from the abnormal oxidation of body fats and oils. Such abnormal oxidation of fats form peroxides, which are, these authors say, "immune system suppressants" and, possibly, cancer-causing agents. They further state that macrophages, a type of white blood cell instrumental in attacking and killing harmful bacteria and other invading "enemies," do not function fully and are "inhibited in the presence of peroxidized fats." Selenium, then, contributes to the breakdown of fats and other body chemicals while allowing the immune system's fighting cells to mobilize efficiently.

Although there has been little research on effects of selenium deficiency in humans, animal research studies show a definite connection to an accelerated aging process and immune system weakening. In *Jane Brody's Nutrition Book* the author reports that it is known that deaths from cancer and high blood pressure are greater in those parts of the country where selenium content of local drinking water is lower.

Megadosing on selenium or any other mineral is not advisable, since they can accumulate to toxic levels in the body or alter a vital process. The National Academy of Sciences' National Research Council established figures for the recommended daily allowance of selenium at .05–.02 mg. In their experimental formula used for themselves and not advised for pregnant women, Pearson and Shaw supplemented their diet with 250 *micrograms,* which is about ten times the RDA dosage. I have heard of cases of women with endometriosis who have taken 50–100 *micrograms* per day, along with vitamins E and C, immediately before and during menstruation, and noted positive benefits, most notably, greater relief from pelvic pain.

Best selection of foods with selenium: This mineral is present in seafood, whole-grain cereals, and garlic. Higher fat foods such as egg yolk and whole milk also contain selenium, but you would be better advised to avoid these sources, since they tend to affect endometriosis sufferers adversely.

VITAMINS: WHAT YOU NEED TO FEEL AT YOUR BEST

In 1911, while searching for a cure for beriberi, the nutritional plague of his day, Polish chemist Casimir Funk described the substance he had isolated as its cause as a "vital amine," or essential amino acid. What he found was soon to be called thiamine, later discovered to be part of a complex group of organic compounds known as vitamins, which are essential for proper bodily growth and maintenance of bodily functions.

Many vitamins cannot be manufactured by the body and must be obtained from food sources or vitamin supplements. Pearson and Shaw, as well as the late Nobel Prize-winning scientist Linus Pauling and many other doctors, researchers, and nutritionists, proselytize for vitamin megadosing—espousing the "more is better, but with caution" school of thought. Practitioners of the macrobiotic diet, in contrast, believe that vitamin supplements are entirely unnecessary, if not detrimental to health. In all, the fact is that if we added up all the vitamins we required per day, the total would just fill about *one-eighth of a teaspoon.* It's not much, but at the same time, it's everything.

My own feeling is to dose wisely. Every woman's needs are different, depending on her diet, her weight, and most important, her general health. In devising guidelines for the woman with endometriosis, we first have to examine the two types of vitamins and how they are best absorbed in the body. Some vitamins are water-soluble and others are fat-soluble.

Water-soluble vitamins include C and the eleven vitamins constituting the B group. These vitamins tend to be used up or washed freely out of your system and should be replenished on a daily basis. Vitamin C is particularly susceptible to breakdown: it can be lost in citrus juice, for example, just by exposure to the air, or it can be destroyed in vegetables by cooking. Fat-soluble vitamins, such as A, D, E, and K, are relatively more resistant to heat and require the aid of fat before they can be absorbed into the body. These vitamins are not flushed from the system but are stored in body fat and drawn upon when needed.

Endometriosis sufferers need the following vitamins most specifically in their diet either to help build immune systems or to help regulate hormonal levels and lessen nervous fatigue.

VITAMIN GUIDELINES

Before taking vitamins, examine this checklist to be sure you will get the most from them:

• Are you on any medication? Ask your doctor if any increase of your vitamin (or mineral) intake will alter the effects of the drug you are taking, or if the vitamin will combine with the drug in such a way as to render blood or urine tests abnormal.

• Don't sacrifice sensible eating and rely on vitamin pills to provide what your body needs.

• You will get the most benefit from the important B and C water-soluble vitamins right after a meal. If you are taking a high dose of vitamin C in separate tablets, you might do better to divide it into smaller doses and take it a few times during the day. Your body chemistry may be such that you cannot absorb a higher dose and just eliminate the excess in your urine.

• The fat-soluble vitamins (A, D, E, K) are best taken either during or right after a meal that has *some* dietary fat. This helps their absorption in the small intestine.

• Stay within the dosage guidelines. Megadosing without supervision can be costly to your health.

The B Vitamins

The "complex" B's are actually a group of eleven separate but interrelated vitamins. They are vitamin B_1 (thiamine), B_2 (riboflavin), B_6 (pyridoxine), B_3 (niacin), B_{12} (cobalamin), pantothenic acid, biotin, folic acid, choline, inositol, and PABA (para-aminobenzoic acid). *All* B vitamins are intimately involved with the breakdown of carbohydrate, protein, and fat in the body, powering the mechanisms that release energy to the muscle cells. B_6 has been shown to influence the release of the brain's neurotransmitters dopamine and serotonin and may be the most critical vitamin for women. These neurotransmitters regulate mood, and a lack may cause a sense of agitation or depression. Folic acid and B_{12} are instrumental in red blood cell production, and red blood cells, in turn, transport oxygen to muscles. Research on choline points to some evidence that this vitamin is linked to brain chemistry and may be a factor in memory retention. Physical activity, alcohol, refined sugar, birth control pills, and emotional stress deplete B vitamins, and since they aren't stored in the body, the more active or under stress you are, the more you need.

These vitamins not only regulate the menstrual cycle but are also crucial for the well-being of women with endometriosis and have been known to help lessen symptoms of PMS. To begin, B vitamins are implicated in liver function and in the synthesis of estrogen. This hormone is broken by the liver into a more benign form, called estriol, which will not make cells proliferate. Undegraded estrogen, called estradiol, is closely linked to endometriosis as well as to cases of fibrocystic disease and breast cancer, uterine fibroids, and heavy menstrual flow. If a woman's diet is poor in B complex vitamins, liver function is impaired and more estradiol enters the system, causing greater endometrial inflammation.

Women who are taking oral contraceptives, are pregnant and/or lactating, and those with endometriosis are all subject to greater B complex needs because of altered or unbalanced hormonal states. An intake of these vitamins should help to elevate moods, control fluid retention, and improve hair and skin quality.

Dr. Robert Atkins, author of the widely acclaimed *Dr. Atkins' Diet Revolution* and its sequel, *Dr. Atkins' New Medicine,* and founder of the Atkins Center for Complementary Medicine in New York, discussed with me his findings on the treatment of endometriosis and vitamin regimens. "We see many patients at the center who have endometriosis, fibrocystic breast disease, and uterine fibroids," he said. "We seek to lower their estrogen based on a sugarless diet, the use of certain B vitamins, especially choline and inositol, and methionine, which is an amino acid. These are all lipotropic agents, or substances that attract and absorb fats. Without choline, fatty deposits would accumulate in the liver. Inositol and methionine work with choline to prevent this from happening. The tendency to produce estrogen is counteracted by these liver-stimulating factors. We give about 1,500 milligrams of each of these three nutrients.

"Conversely," he added, "folic acid and PABA are two nutrients that can *increase* estrogen activity. Since dietary folic acid is found in green vegetables, I would not go so far as to recommend cutting down on it. Rather, I would concentrate on building up every other B vitamin, within reasonable and safe dosages."

Dosage: B complex is best taken in a balanced-formula pill. Taking an overload of one of these vitamins may increase the need for the others. Since these vitamins are water-soluble, you'll do best to take them with meals. A full stomach will also offset any side effects of the dosage, such as mild nausea. To keep mood and hormones balanced harmoniously, endometriosis sufferers should begin with a 100-mg B complex tablet, with an additional 50–200 mg of B_6. From the two weeks before the menstrual cycle, increase vitamin B_6 intake to 500 mg and take it along with B complex and magnesium tablets. This combination should help reduce estrogen overloading. It's a good idea not to take a high-dosage vitamin C supplement at the same time you are taking the B's. Vitamin C in large quantities tends to destroy B_{12}.

Best selection of foods with B vitamins: These critically important vitamins are often sacrificed by overcooking, canning, overprocessing, and long-term storage—an unfortunate byproduct of the modern food industry. It may not be an intentional disservice, but nevertheless, we are sometimes consuming prepackaged foods that are poor in B complex vitamins when they should be naturally B complex rich. Strive, then, for the freshest food products. To benefit most, the best sources are liver, brewer's yeast, whole grains (wheat bran, rice bran, oatmeal), soybeans, peanuts, peas, lima beans, dark leafy vegetables, tuna, turkey, veal, asparagus, walnuts, and raw pecans.

Vitamin C

Among its many properties, vitamin C builds and maintains collagen, the basis of the most abundant connective tissue that joins and cements the body's cells, in skin, bones, and teeth. Energy levels can be increased when this vitamin, in part, cues the liver to release glycogen as glucose into the bloodstream. Vitamin C has a well-deserved reputation as stimulator of the immune system to help promote healing and provide greater resistance to disease. Research is being done to relate vitamin C to an ability to block the development of cancer-causing chemicals such as nitrosamines in the digestive system.

Dosage: Every woman's needs will be different for vitamin C, but it's a good idea for a sufferer of endometriosis to increase the amount of this vitamin. Begin with 1,000 mg a day during the month, then increase your dosage to 1,500 mg from the midcycle through the menstrual period. Take larger amounts of vitamin C in two to four doses over the day. If you megadose on this vitamin and take *over* 4,000 mg of it per day, you may develop diarrhea or find you are urinating more frequently.

Best selection of foods with vitamin C: Citrus fruits are usually the first choice among foods high in this vitamin, but endometriosis sufferers may do well to cut down on them. While citrus fruit is rich in vitamin C, it also contains substances called bioflavinoids, which may mimic the effects of estrogen, possibly adding to the discomforts of endometriosis flare-ups. During particularly stressful menstrual periods when you are most symptomatic, limit or avoid oranges, grapefruit, lemons, limes, and tangerines (or their juices), strawberries, and cantaloupe, and get the vitamin C you need from supplements and vegetable sources. A few excellent choices are brussels sprouts, green or red peppers, collard greens, and potatoes. A portion of kale or mustard greens (about three-fourths of a cup) has two to three times as much vitamin C as a whole orange.

Vitamin A

The first fat-soluble vitamin to be discovered, vitamin A is found in carotene, a yellow dye that occurs abundantly in yellow, orange, red, or dark green leafy vegetables. Vitamin A, synthesized from carotene, is nutritionally significant. It is an excellent immune system booster. It has the capability of increasing the size of the thymus gland (the master gland of the immune system). As reported in *Life Extension,* one study showed that the thymus may lose up to 95 percent of its vitamin A content following an injury, which, the authors theorize, is why infections so easily set in after physical traumas.

The carotenes have been scrutinized in the last decade for their potential as great healing agents, and beta-carotene, in particular, has been tested in the treatment of cancers. This last point is still controversial, as some scientists think that beta-carotene may stimulate cancer growth, not retard it. But we are speaking of megadoses. For our purposes, vitamin A or beta-carotene supplements may be of some benefit. Besides their critical role in maintaining normal vision and preventing night blindness, vitamin A is also essential for maintaining the mucous membranes that line the eyes and the gastrointestinal, respiratory, and genitourinary tracts.

Since symptoms of endometriosis can weaken the immune system, vitamin A dosage can help strengthen the body's ability to fight back. The American Cancer Society, in fact, recommends an increase in the daily intake of both vitamins A and C to strengthen the immune system.

Dosage: Vitamin A taken too enthusiastically can be toxic, since it is stored in the liver. Beta-carotene, however, is not converted into vitamin A unless the body requires it, and you cannot suffer from toxic levels of it. You do best to take 5,000 units of vitamin A in combination with other vitamins. If you are also taking vitamins C and E—both immune system builders—this amount of A should be sufficient. If you choose beta-carotene, take one 10,000-unit capsule a day.

Best selection of foods with vitamin A: This is one case where you can discern a correlation between the carotene content by the *color* of the food. Green cabbage pales in vitamin A content in comparison with carrots, apricots, yellow squash, pumpkin, cantaloupe, turnip tops, beets and beet greens, and broccoli, which are all excellent sources of this vitamin. Animal foods with vitamin A are liver, egg yolk, butter, and fortified margarines, to name a few. By far the best source is an ounce and a half of parsley with 4,200 units of the vitamin.

Vitamin E

There is somewhat of a mystique about this fat-soluble vitamin in terms of its curative powers, antiaging factors, increased oxygen-carrying capacities, immune system strengthening powers, and its implications in production of sex hormones in men and women. While it has been hailed by many as the miracle vitamin of the 1980s, its abilities have been only partially determined. Vitamin E is related to the sex hormones chemically, and it was first discovered in a study on antisterility factors.

Vitamin E reputedly helps oxygenate the blood by increasing hemoglobin's ability to carry oxygen. It is also able to minimize the oxidation of vitamin A and carotene in the intestine, thereby prolonging the effect of vitamin A. Vitamin E is gaining favor as an "antiaging" vitamin among believers who say that it can delay the breakdown of cells. A number of studies have been conducted among women with fibrocystic disease to see if vitamin E had any effect on the curing or halting of this condition. As yet, there is no conclusive evidence that this vitamin can be taken as a preventive for fibrocystic disease.

Dosage: Working in tandem with vitamins A and C, vitamin E taken in 400 to 800 units a day will strengthen the immune system and help prolong the effects of vitamin A. Keep this level up through the month.

Best selection of foods with vitamin E: Wheat germ, nuts, whole grains, and rice germ are the most potent sources of vitamin E. There is some concentration of it in green leafy vegetables and the legumes.

Vitamin K

This vitamin is essential to forming prothrombin, a blood-clotting chemical. The vitamin was discovered by a Danish doctor who found that a *"koagulations* vitamin" was necessary to promote normal clotting factors and prevent any fatal hemorrhaging.

Vitamin K is partially manufactured by bacterial action in the intestines, but bile salts from the liver are necessary for its absorption into the body from the intestines. (In fact, newborns are given injections of this vitamin at birth to prevent bleeding disorders. Until they are a few days old, there is no intestinal bacterial action to help produce K naturally.) Antibiotics will most interfere with the synthesis of the vitamin. Some physicians prescribe a vitamin K regimen for a week preceding scheduled surgery, but this is not necessary in every case. Your doctor will determine if you need an extra dose of K prior to surgery.

Dosage: Vitamin K is stored in the liver, but only in minute amounts. The daily requirement of vitamin K is now set at 10 mg. If you tend to bleed heavily during your menstrual cycle, increase your dose of vitamin K to 20 mg a day for those days.

Best selection of foods with vitamin K: Green leafy plants like cabbage, kale, collard greens, and spinach are excellent sources of this vitamin. Pork liver is high in this vitamin, but it is also high in cholesterol. To keep friendly bacteria actively producing this vitamin in your intestine, you may opt to take acidophilus tablets, which have no calories, instead of yogurt or acidophilus milk.

THE ENDOMETRIOSIS DIET

The goal of this plan is to structure your dietary intake and relieve or prevent some of the more disabling symptoms of endometriosis. The plan has been designed to work over the long run to *decrease* your estrogen level and *stabilize* hormones, *increase* energy, *alleviate* extreme menstrual cramping, and *work as a calmative* for emotional and physical distress. You will need to analyze your own case and judge your own needs, following the calendar in chapter 6 to chart mood changes, bleeding patterns, and pelvic pain.

This diet is a basic regimen that stresses low-fat, low-sugar, low-salt, low-cholesterol, low-dairy-product intake, which is especially advisable during the menstrual cycle and for at least ten days preceding it. I have used it successfully with my own patients and found it can help them. *This is not a weight-loss diet,* although you might indeed stabilize your weight or lose a pound or two. If you are unable to stay on the diet for ten days of the month, try to follow the suggestions on alternate days. It will help to work as a "cleansing" or balancing diet.

Diet Guidelines

• If you are inclined toward hypoglycemia, you will want to keep blood sugar at a steady level and avoid roller coaster peaks and valleys of hypoglycemia. One way of controlling symptoms of hypoglycemia is to avoid sugar in the form of candies and rich desserts. (More on this very shortly.) Instead, develop the habit of eating smaller, more frequent meals—of the kind that will soon follow. This could entail a total of six small meals a day rather than two or three larger ones. Frequent and balanced small meals can help you avoid candy bars or sweetened sodas or fruit drinks to substitute for missed larger "main" meals. A highly concentrated amount of sugar may cause an insulin rush and a subsequent drop in blood sugar, resulting in a feeling of fatigue, depression, and irritability.

• Discover substitutes. The endometriosis recovery diet may be asking you to give up (or limit) some foods you especially love, such as grilled-cheese sandwiches, chocolate milk, avocados, large quantities of fruit juice, coffee, junk food, and alcoholic beverages. They may taste good, but they are not good for what ails you now. The ingredients that go into these foods include high-fat, high-cholesterol oils such as hydrogenated oils or lard, high-fat cheese and other dairy products, cocoa, an excess of fruit, caffeine, highly processed salt-laden fast food, and alcohol. For at least ten days of the month, or *about* five days prior to menstruation and during the five days of the menstrual cycle, lower your intake of these foods and use equally nutritious and tasty alternates.

To help cut back on *dairy* products, use soy milk, soy cheese, tofu cakes, soy-based mayonnaise, and if you have a craving for dessert, even tofu "ice cream" (one brand is Ice Bean) made from this versatile and healthful bean. Soy products, slightly bland from lack of flavor-making fat (though soybeans do contain a very low amount of poly-unsaturated fat) and no sugar content, are nutritious, nearly complete high-protein foods that are naturally low in calories. One cup of soybean milk, for example, contains only 87 calories. Tofu, which can be substituted for cottage cheese and used in a wide variety of recipes, is also low-calorie (about 72 calories per four-ounce cake). A four-ounce cake of tofu also has 128 grams of calcium, whereas four ounces of 2-percent-fat cottage cheese contains only 77 grams of calcium.

• Keep salt intake at the desirable "half a teaspoon or less per day" requirement for the target period; use salt substitutes or prepared spice mixes like Spike or Vegal. Aromatic garlic, reputed to be beneficial to health as a blood purifier, is a good choice to add to salad dressings and fish dishes. Spices and herbs such as rosemary, ginger, and red pepper are all thought by herbalists to be tonifiers to the reproductive system.

• Reduce sugar intake. This is probably the most difficult guideline of all to follow, since sugar cravings strike a large proportion of women premenstrually and during the menstrual cycle. Sugar also supplies psychological comfort for some women during stressful times. Paradoxically, processed sugars, or disaccharides, can be candy-coated trouble and induce conditions like *hypoglycemia*.

Hypoglycemia is a condition in which higher insulin levels cause blood sugar levels to fluctuate rapidly. One of insulin's functions is to clear the blood of excess sugar. Concentrated, or simple, sugars trigger an overproduction of this hormone, which, in turn, clears the blood of too much sugar. High insulin levels also may be caused by an imbalance of brain hormones and neurotransmitters or an imbalance of estrogen and progesterone—or all of these factors—causing the body's blood sugar level to plummet. A high insulin/low blood sugar ratio may signal a possible attack of hypoglycemia in men as well as women. It can be characterized by a feeling of "depletion," exhaustion, the onset of a headache, which is answered by a physical craving for sugar, usually consumed in its most accessible form—candy, brownies, ice cream. Since sugar travels quickly to the bloodstream,

VITAMIN CHART

Vitamin	Good Sources	Functions
A	Yellow, orange, dark green vegetables and fruits (carrots, yellow squash, cantaloupe, apricots, spinach, broccoli)	Assists in function of immune and reproductive systems; needed to prevent night blindness and in formation of hair, skin, mucous membranes and teeth
B_1 (Thiamine)	Enriched cereals and grains (e.g. brown rice, wheat germ, oatmeal) beans (soy, lima), oysters, artichokes,	Essential in certain metabolic processes; helps transmit nerve impulses
B_2 (Riboflavin)	Whole grains, nuts, liver, dark green leafy vegetables, mushrooms, enriched bread	Similar functions to B_1; helps maintain mucous membranes
B_3 (Niacin)	Tuna, poultry, dried nuts and beans, peas, rice bran	Works with B_1 and B_2 in helping production of energy in cells
B_6 (Pyridoxine)	Leafy vegetables, lentils, tuna, bananas, whole grain	Antioxidant; helps in formation of red blood cells; transports amino acids; may protect against artery damage by helping body utilize fats
B_{12} (Cobalamin)	Only available from animal sources (beef, fish, milk, oysters)	Helps formation of genetic material, aids in building red blood cells
Biotin	Soy flour, beans, egg yolk, cauliflower, liver	Aids in release of energy from carbohydrates
Pantothenic Acid	Whole grain cereals, nuts, eggs, liver, dark green vegetables	Important role in energy production; antistress vitamin; helps in formation of hormones
Folic Acid	Dark green vegetables, wheat germ, watermelon, asparagus, cantaloupe	Helps synthesize genetic material and red blood cells
Choline	Milk, lecithin, peanut butter, wheat germ; most often produced in the body	Strengthens immune system; reputedly enhances memory

134

Vitamin	Good Sources	Functions
Inositol	Brewer's yeast; cantaloupe, oranges, raisins	Can aid in fat metabolism
PABA (Para-amino-benzoic Acid)	Yeast, blackstrap molasses, whole grains, potatoes	Helps fight infection; an antioxidant, works with B_6 to prevent certain anemias; may help slow aging in skin when used topically in creams
C	Citrus fruits, cantaloupe, brussels sprouts, green or red peppers, collard greens, kale, mustard greens	Stimulator of the immune system; builds and maintains collagen; helps maintain health of teeth, gums capillaries and bones
D	Sunlight produces it in skin; egg yolk, salmon, liver	Helps in formation and maintenance of bones and teeth; needed in absorption of calcium and phosphorus
E	Vegetable oils, wheat germ, whole grain cereals, green leafy vegetables	Protects vitamin A and essential fatty acids from oxidation; aids in formation of red blood cells
K	Green leafy vegetables, potatoes, cauliflower	Aids in blood-clotting factors to prevent hemorrhaging

the unpleasant symptoms of hypoglycemia seem to be quelled by an immediate sense of relief. However, within half an hour to an hour, blood chemistry will change radically: the high insulin level will increase once again as blood sugar levels fall.

Rather than eating foods laden with refined sugar or overprocessed carbohydrates (white bread, cake, pie, etc.), choose fresh vegetables, fibrous fruits on a limited basis (like an apple a day), small amounts of whole grains (as in a bran muffin), and some protein at regular intervals to keep blood sugar constant.

• Reduce caffeine. I've had patients with endometriosis who claim to drink six or more cups of coffee a day and never suffer any effects of excessive caffeine intake other than frequent urination. Why? Habitual users of caffeine in the form of coffee, cola, and/or chocolate can build up a tolerance to it. The woman with endometriosis, however, is wise to eliminate or reduce caffeine in her diet *every* day, not just during the week before her menstrual cycle begins. Caffeine may aggravate her condition in a number of ways. While it can spark thought processes and induce wakefulness, it is similar to simple sugars in that it can cause insulin to pour into the blood, creating a drop in blood sugar levels.

Caffeine in larger quantities has been linked to the development of fibrocystic disease, the most common noncancerous condition of the breast. Studies continue to investigate the connection between chemicals known as methylxanthines, which are found in various edible forms in coffee, chocolate, and tea, and the growth of these breast lumps. As yet, there is no answer as to why breast lumps grow in *some* women who use caffeine, other than the theory that estrogen and progesterone receptors in breast tissue are sensitive to these biochemicals. Other women have no such problem. Women with fibrocystic disease often report swelling and tenderness of the breast premenstrually and during menstruation.

The FDA regards caffeine as a *drug,* not just a harmless ingredient in a soft drink. In addition to the investigation of caffeine's role in fibrocystic breast disease, there is research into some types of pancreatic disorders and caffeine's effects on the rate of miscarriage and birth defects.

Caffeine drinks produce a jolt of energy—hence their popularity. Caffeine is not just a drug, but an ergogenic, a substance that provides energy. Like alcohol, it speeds through the blood-brain barrier, quickly stimulating the central nervous system, accelerating the heartbeat, and sharpening coordination. It can increase muscle efficiency (some experienced runners have a cup of strong coffee before a race) and it changes respiration and metabolic rates. But remember, it can also, like sugar, set up conditions that encourage an attack of hypoglycemia.

Caffeine is also found in nonherbal tea, over-the-counter PMS preparations like Midol, and analgesics like Anacin. In any of these forms, caffeine will interfere with the absorption of B vitamins, causing, among other conditions, a sense of fatigue as well as triggering a greater secretion of stomach acid, producing "heartburn." If you cannot give up caffeine entirely, limit yourself to one drink of your choice a day. Switch to coffee substitutes like Postum or Pero or any number of caffeine-free teas and coffees as often as you can. Although dedicated chocoholics won't concede its victory as a reasonable choco-late substitute, carob is close enough to the real thing. Carob is fat- and caffeine-free and has about one-third the calories of chocolate. Sold in health food stores, you can purchase it in as many forms as chocolate—powdered, syrup, candy bits, and so on.

How Will You Feel on This Diet?

Some women will have an immediate sense of well-being after only a week on the diet. Others may not respond as quickly. One reason is that ovaries are sensitive to dietary changes, especially to an increase in B complex vitamins and a withdrawal or lessening of fats and sugar. The liver will continue to degrade estrogen to estriol, but the ovaries may respond in a contrary fashion. Instead of estrogen output being controlled by diet, the ovaries are, so to speak, tricked into believing that they are lagging behind in producing the hormone and may speed up production for a few days. Eventually, however, the body adjusts to a different dietary mode. The endometriosis recovery diet should foster a sense of relief and well-being. Because of it, some women may be able to free themselves from painkillers, tranquilizers, and, in selected cases, hormone treatments.

Breakfast

This is often the most problematic meal of the day, since many women do not like to eat breakfast or don't have the time. I strongly urge you to begin the day with some nutrition, to keep blood sugar levels stabilized. A small bowl of *whole-grain* cereal with half a cup of soy milk (or low-fat milk) supplies carbohydrates, protein, and some calcium from the soy. Hot cereal such as oatmeal, cooked with a tablespoon of raisins, is good, too. Half a grapefruit or, better, a noncitrus fruit like a small banana adds sufficient sugar. Limit egg intake to one or two a week. These should be boiled or poached. Choose *organic* fertilized eggs, available at many supermarkets now. They taste the same as the standard egg, but contain less cholesterol. If you don't have cereal or one egg, have a high-fiber bran muffin or one or two slices of toasted whole-wheat bread with half an apple.

This menu offers protein, carbohydrates, and minimum fat and is fairly low in calories. It begins the program to lower disruptive hormone levels in women with endometriosis while simultaneously supplying energy.

If you want a cup of coffee or tea (or any drink with caffeine), have it at breakfast time, rather than later in the day. Caffeine takes about half an hour before it supplies its "kick," and close to four hours before its effect wears off. One result of caffeine on the drop in blood sugar level is a sense of hunger. By the time you feel this, you should be ready for lunch, which, like dinner, should consist of foods that will maintain a steady blood sugar level.

Lunch

The midday meal should feature a small portion of high-protein food, such as water-packed tuna or canned salmon with a tossed green salad and a low-fat, low-salt dressing, preferably made with not more than two tablespoons of safflower or walnut oil. If you prepare your lunch at home and take it to your place of work, you may add a tablespoon of soy-based mayonnaise and chopped onion to the tuna or salmon. Alternates are white-meat turkey, cold seafood salad, or a cold tossed pasta salad made with diced fresh vegetables. Homemade (or low-salt) vegetable soups or bean soups (like lentil) are a good bet, along with one slice of whole-wheat bread. Other choices include steamed vegetable plate, a plain baked potato, and bean salad. For dessert, have the other half of the apple left from breakfast.

If you want to have cottage cheese or any other dairy product, high-citrus fruits, or sugary desserts, have them at the midday meal. "Fat attack" cravings, if you cannot resist them, are best indulged (in moderation) at lunch rather than at dinner. A number of studies on metabolism and diet indicate why: it is now thought that weight gain is a likelier possibility from calories consumed later in the day than earlier.

Dinner

For dinner, try to stress steamed fresh vegetables, such as squash, broccoli, kale, and others rich in B complex and vitamin A, served with a small (six-ounce) portion of fish, very lean meat if you are a confirmed lover of red meat, or poultry. You may also try a vegetarian dinner of brown rice, steamed vegetables (such as broccoli, carrot chunks, white turnip or parsnips, yellow squash or pumpkin or kale), a cup of cooked beans (such as soybeans, lentils, chick-peas, or small red beans). For dessert, indulge in a small portion of soy-based ice cream, fruit, or unbuttered, unsalted popcorn, popped, if possible, by air heating, not oil.

Snacking

You want to do what you can nutritionally to help alleviate cramps, pelvic pain, bloating, and fluctuating blood sugar levels. It's best to try this diet for two days to see how you feel. If you tend toward PMS along with problems associated with endometriosis, or if you are feeling hungry, you may want to eat a piece of bran or corn muffin, rice cakes, half a banana, or a handful of strawberries every three hours or so, to help manage any blood sugar imbalances.

I firmly believe that these nutritional and stress-reducing guidelines can make a positive difference in reducing pain and extreme hormone fluctuations for many women. Keeping to the diet for at least three menstrual cycles will give you the information you need about how your body responds to these dietary changes. After that, you can make adjustments that will ease you through the difficult cycles of endometriosis. Increasing exercise and giving yourself time for well-deserved rest and tranquillity can only aid in suppressing the disease.

Endometriosis is a complex of symptoms that occurs in phases and strikes each woman differently. Until science can pinpoint the precise cause of endometriosis, with *all* its possible variables, you can use this natural approach to seeing some improvement and healing your body. If you still experience incapacitating symptoms, you might be a candidate for further medical treatment of a specific nature: hormone treatments. Chapter 10 discusses these in detail.

Hormone Treatments

THIRTY years ago, diagnosis and management of endometriosis were partially obscured by limited knowledge. Laparoscopy did not exist then, laser microsurgery was more the dream of hopeful futurists; nor was there the range of sophisticated studies of endometriosis focusing on every aspect of it from pain control to actually creating the disease in the laboratory.

Hormone treatment for endometriosis tended to be concentrated on high doses of progestin, diethylstilbestrol (synthetic female sex hormones, also called DES), or methyltestosterone (synthetic male sex hormones), but they proved to cause grave side effects, with only small improvement in helping to cure endometriosis. The rationale for prescribing these hormones was based on two known facts about the disease: endometriosis tended to (1) regress or disappear for a time after pregnancy or (2) regress or disappear after menopause.

The reasons these "natural cures" tend to work are these: pregnancy gives the body a rest from retrograde menstruation, menstrual cramps, and the growth of endometrial masses; menopause brings the female reproductive cycle to a close so that not only does menstruation cease but hormones drop permanently to a level that cannot sustain endometriosis. In prescribing diethylstilbestrol or progestin-only supplements, the body was put into a stage of *pseudopregnancy*; in giving methyltestosterone, the estrogen level was manipulated to fool the body into *pseudomenopause*.

A more drastic solution in severe cases of endometriosis was hysterectomy—that is, the removel of what was thought to be the source of the problem. Age was not a factor in performing hysterectomy; young childless women were castrated along with older women who had already borne children. But, as it was later discovered (and as I will explain in chapter 13), *hysterectomy does not cure endometriosis*.

Hormones are subtle but powerful chemicals. Since the 1950s, medicine has been energetically searching for the answer to endometriosis within these substances. The ideology behind prescribing hormones today is essentially the same as in yesteryear: create pseudopregnancy or pseudomenopause, and the disease can be halted, prevented, or "melted away." Since the days of Stilbestrol (diethylstilbestrol), however, we have learned a lot about what will work and what will not. Despite this, a number of myths still exist concerning the link between hormones and endometriosis, so let's begin there.

CAN PREGNANCY CURE ENDOMETRIOSIS?

"I got my period when I was ten years old. Two years later, I had exploratory surgery because of ovarian cysts," Paula, a twenty-five-year-old mother of two wrote to me from Minnesota. Just beginning her career in sales, Paula is facing a crossroads in medical care of her endometriosis. Her letter continues: "Over the years, I've been diagnosed as having a spasmodic condition, and told I was a nervous person whenever I complained of menstrual cramps. I know now that it was PMS, in part.

"I was married at eighteen, and pregnant when I was nineteen. I felt okay until three months after my son was born," Paula continued. "My gynecologist told me I had an enlarged uterus due to an infection. He put me on antibiotics. Then I conceived again and had a difficult pregnancy. I went into labor for two days. My cervix didn't want to open up. I ended up with a cesarean section. Six months later, the pain came back again. My doctor put me in the hospital for a laparoscopy. He found extensive endometriosis and so much scar tissue on my right ovary that it had to be removed. He said it was just a matter of time before I'd need a hysterectomy. I went to another doctor and he recommended birth control pills. I just can't take them because they make me dizzy, headachy, and bloated. He also said that my left ovary was adhered to my uterus from endometriosis. He said that if I can't take the Pill, I should get pregnant again and breast-feed for a year, and that then I might be okay again. Why would I get better if I had a third child when the other two pregnancies didn't help? My husband has been wonderful through all of this, but he's as confused about all this as I am. Should I just give in and have a hysterectomy? I am desperate. We would appreciate any advice."

Paula's story is a classic example of a woman whose condition should have been medically managed with hormones, beginning in her early teens. In her case, oral contraceptives taken during those years might have halted the spread of the disease that clearly took root when she was very young. Instead, like thousands and thousands of other women before her, Paula has been misguided into believing that pregnancy cures endometriosis. The "scientific" proof behind this theory is a commonsense observation: doctors noted that endometriosis often improved after a woman had a child, and that women who had one child after the other in relatively rapid succession had fewer signs of endometriosis and complained less of symptoms of the disease than women who were childless. If you are pregnant, you do not menstruate for nine months; breast feeding continues the cessation of menstruation and regulates fluctuating hormones on a monthly basis. You can see how doctors might suggest pregnancy as a cure. It provides a woman's body with what is familiarly called a pelvic rest. Actually, the fact that Paula was able to conceive a second time gives some credence to this theory: after her first child and a pelvic rest, endometriosis was suppressed enough that she was able to conceive again. However, since endometriosis often causes infertility, it is a catch-22: a woman is told to get pregnant to improve her endometriosis, but endometriosis prevents her from getting pregnant.

A number of other things happen during pregnancy that led doctors to conclude that pregnancy was, if not a panacea, then a means to an eventual cure through self-healing. Other than normalizing hormone levels, amenorrhea to prevent retrograde menstruation, and the additional pelvic rest gained by breast feeding, doctors believed that the stretching of pelvic organs during pregnancy was beneficial. If the uterus is stuck with adhesions or is tilted backward, pregnancy will cause the uterus to expand and lift itself upward into a nearly normal position in the pelvis. This might "naturally" free some of the adhesions, reducing pain. After childbirth, however, the uterus might go back into the retroverted position and adhesions can re-form. This healthy and natural stretching of organs explains why some women feel somewhat better after childbirth. Nonetheless, *pregnancy does not cure endometriosis, although it might slow down its progression.*

Another problem for Paula was a high prolactin level, which is associated with breast feeding, and, in fact, *may* be a factor contributing to premenstrual syndrome. I have treated many women like Paula who suffer from both PMS and endometriosis—two conditions related to menstruation which can coexist. Sometimes the symptoms of PMS can be confused with those of endometriosis, especially pain during ovulation (mittelschmerz). It is important for such women who may also have PMS to note that the prolactin level fluctuates on a daily basis, but that it peaks during ovulation. The level is lower in the first half of the menstrual cycle than the second.

A hormone triggered by the pituitary gland, prolactin, stimulates the production and secretion of breast milk. Obviously, prolactin levels will be higher in nursing mothers. Interestingly, this hormone can increase in response to suction on the breast as well as any kind of emotional stress *unrelated* to pregnancy and nursing. Research shows that prolactin reaches *higher* levels at different points in the menstrual cycles of women who have PMS. When prolactin levels rise, a variety of symptoms can appear. Even a slightly increased level of prolactin could induce PMS, since this hormone inhibits the fluctuations of the brain hormones FSH and LH, which affect production of estrogen and progesterone. Moderately high prolactin levels can influence hormone production even further, by altering the menstrual cycle.

Other associated effects are weight gain and PMS symptoms, which are related to an excess of estrogen. Very high prolactin levels can cause amenorrhea (which can lead to infertility) or (in nursing women) no menstruation and galactorrhea, or leakage of milk from the nipples. High prolactin levels may signal the presence of microadenomas, small tumors in the pituitary gland, but this is rarer.

High prolactin levels have been treated with Parlodel (bromocriptine), a drug that is known to block production of this hormone and stop milk secretion (when it exists) while reestablishing the synchronized fluctuations of the brain and the female hormones. Although bromocriptine has helped some women with PMS, an equal number of women studied have not benefited from its use. In my practice, I have found that prolactin levels may sometimes contribute to PMS. In Paula's case, it is possible that she is more sensitive to this hormone during her normal menstrual cycles and while breast feeding.

Paula is only twenty-five years old and in her prime reproductive years. She should not have a hysterectomy. I must stress that removal of the uterus does *not* guarantee a cure for endometriosis. Remember, one of the insidious qualities of this disease is that it sprays renegade cells into the abdominal cavity. These cells are living tissue, surviving on a host organ, "fed" by the female hormones. Removal of the uterus alone merely removes the source of endometrial tissue capable of implantation. *Unless the ovaries are also removed,* causing menopause, endometriosis can remain active. *Hormone replacement therapy,* or estrogen supplementation, often administered to ease the suddenness of menopause, only serves to restimulate the growth of the disease in many cases.

It is my belief that at this point in her life, Paula will benefit most from the endometriosis diet and stress-reduction techniques in conjunction with a program of Danocrine, the "antihormone," which I will discuss in detail in a moment.

ARE BIRTH CONTROL PILLS THE TREATMENT OF CHOICE?

I have received countless letters asking me about the efficacy of birth control pills in either curing or preventing endometriosis. The range of ages of the affected women has been from fourteen years old to forty-six years old. At one time, oral contraceptives were thought by some of the medical establishment to be the answer for curing endometriosis. After a program of pills, doctors believed, the endometriosis would be deactivated and the body would be healthy enough to prevent a recurrence. Yet I receive letters like this one:

"Besides myself, I have three friends and a sister-in-law with endometriosis and I think we have tried everything," wrote Vicki, a thirty-four-year-old who has recently left her job at a travel agency in Alaska to care for her newborn son. "We have had eleven operations between us, we have taken estrogen or progesterone treatments, and now my sister-in-law is on a double dose of birth control pills. She is at the end of her rope and feels worse than ever. I am now on birth control pills for two reasons. The doctor said it will stop the endometriosis from worsening, and my husband and I don't want another child for a few years. Are we putting ourselves in some danger by taking these hormones?"

A New Jersey woman wrote me for advice when the birth control pills she was taking began to affect her badly. Mostly, she complained of psychological effects such as depression, severe headaches, irritability, and even memory lapses. Her doctor insisted she continue on the pills for another two months, or get pregnant. Kathy, who was newly married, told me, "When you have intolerable pain, you believe anyone who says, 'These pills will help.' I took birth control pills when I was eighteen and frightened of becoming pregnant. I had to stop because they made me dizzy and nauseous. Now, ten years later, my doctor gave me Ovral to 'completely suppress' the endometriosis. Guess what? I still have severe pain, but now the pills have given me acne, an increase in body hair, water retention, *and* dizziness and nausea. This is a nightmare. The doctor recommends oral contraceptives until *menopause*. I am only twenty-eight years old and the thought of another fifteen to twenty years of these pills terrifies me!"

The initial theory that supported the use of birth control pills in curing endometriosis is linked to the pregnancy-as-cure theory. Birth control pills work to create a pseudopregnancy, putting the body in a state hormonally where conception cannot occur because the body is tricked into believing that it already is pregnant. Birth control pills contain estrogen and progesterone, the same hormones found in higher concentration among women who are pregnant. Pills may be prescribed in two programs. First, you may take a higher dose pill that more effectively prevents cyclic changes; that is, you take the pills for seven days a week, all month, without stopping for a week. Or you may be on the pills for three weeks, then take a break from them for a week. During the week off the pills, there is a menstrual period, often lighter in flow. The idea of pseudopregnancy improving endometriosis depends on this "trickery." High doses of hormones every day have a feedback mechanism to the brain. They block production of the hypothalamus and pituitary hormones (LH and FSH) that would otherwise stimulate natural hormone production to bring on a menstrual cycle. (See illustration.)

Thousands and thousands of women today are prescribed birth control pills as the main treatment of choice for endometriosis. The pills are being given for an average period of twelve months, to duplicate the nine months of pregnancy and three months of breast feeding. In many cases, women feel better after having taken oral contraceptives, because menstruation and excess prostaglandin production are reduced or eliminated—and they feel less pain. However, the endometriosis tissue *does not melt away*. Instead, the endometrial growths are kept alive because of the high estrogen level. It is possible to give *low-dosage* birth control pills with a low-estrogen formula, for a three-week duration. On these pills, there is less menstrual bleeding. Birth control pills alter the endometrial lining of the uterus, so even if

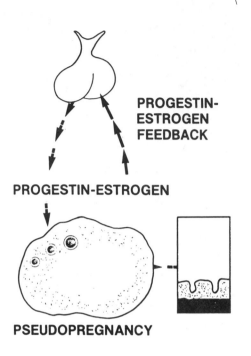

PROGESTIN-
ESTROGEN
FEEDBACK

PROGESTIN-ESTROGEN

PSEUDOPREGNANCY

Pseudopregnancy with Oral Contraceptive Therapy.

Used with permission of Winthrop Pharmaceuticals, New York, NY

there is some retrograde menstruation, these "abnormal" menstrual cells will not cause a buildup of the disease. It is my feeling that low-estrogen birth control pills work on a limited basis for women who have severe menstrual cramps, some signs of premenstrual syndrome, and any evidence of minimal endometriosis. Low-dosage oral contraceptives (less than 35 micrograms of estrogen) have proved beneficial, too, for teenage girls with severe menstrual cramps who are high-risk candidates for developing endometriosis. Since the pills alter endometrial lining and lessen menstrual blood flow, they can reduce the severity and growth of the implants. It is felt that microscopic endometriosis will respond to these pills, but they should not be taken without interruption because it is dangerous to do so, as will be explained shortly.

Birth control pills should not be the first treatment of choice in such cases as Vicki's—women who have documented cases of the disease and who have undergone surgery. The hormones in these pills will not clear up the condition, and can, under certain circumstances, increase the growths due to the estrogen present in the pills.

HOW TO KNOW IF YOU SHOULD NOT TAKE ORAL CONTRACEPTIVES FOR ENDOMETRIOSIS:

Birth control pills carry with them a number of caveats. *Do not* take low- or high-dosage oral contraceptives, even on an experimental basis, to "see how you'll feel," if you suffer from any of the following:

- **fibroid tumors**
- **pelvic masses of unknown type**
- **high blood pressure**
- **diabetes**
- **high cholesterol levels**
- **or, if you are a heavy smoker**

All of these conditions are especially sensitive to estrogen and/or progesterone increase or alteration. You may inadvertently worsen your condition by taking *any* birth control pill formula. If you smoke, and if you are also over thirty-five years old, you may be increasing your chances of cardiovascular disease by taking hormones in this manner.

Although some women with mild endometriosis feel improvement by taking oral contraceptives, often there are side effects that bear close watching, as Kathy mentioned in her letter. Uppermost are:

- water retention or edema
- painful breast engorgement
- headaches and dizziness
- nervousness
- premenstrual syndrome
- the correlation between lipid factors and oral contraceptives

The most important of these side effects is the correlation between lipid factors—triglyceride and cholesterol levels—and contraceptives. Research has shown that the use of oral contraceptives causes changes

147

in the body's levels of HDL (high-density lipoproteins) and LDL (low-density lipoproteins). HDL levels are thought to help prevent heart attack, while LDL may increase the risk of heart attack. Fat metabolism changes while you are on the Pill. LDL increases while you take the synthetic estrogen and progesterone birth control pill.

When LDL increases in the blood, it allows more fat deposits in the blood and narrows the opening (the lumen) in the vascular system, making it easier for blood clots, or embolisms, to form and travel to the brain, heart, or lungs. If you are on the Pill, it is more dangerous to take it every day without interruption for six months or a year than to take it for three weeks of the month, stopping for menstruation,

WHEN TO TAKE BIRTH CONTROL PILLS TO TREAT ENDOMETRIOSIS

Oral contraceptives are *never* the first treatment of choice in the case of *verified* endometriosis. However, there are circumstances when a number of women can benefit from a low-estrogen birth control pill. They are:

• Women in their teens and twenties who suffer from severe menstrual cramps, pelvic pain and discomfort, and pain during ovulation, but who essentially have a *normal* pelvic examination revealing no endometrial masses at all. Such women may take the birth control pill if they are not planning families in the near future.

• Women with *known* endometriosis and/or infertility who have never been cured of the disease with Danocrine and who have successfully conceived and given birth. If they do not want to conceive again right after breast feeding, the birth control pill is recommended to help space childbearing as well as prevent recurring endometriosis.

• Women who have undergone successful treatment of endometriosis with either Danocrine, an analog, or laser surgery and who do not want to conceive right away but will be planning a family in the future.

The birth control pill in these instances should be given in the usual fashion of one pill a day in a usual twenty-eight-day cycle, of which twenty-one days are pills with active ingredients and seven days are placebos.

which is a more normal cyclic pattern. The body then has a chance to normalize during the week before starting on another dose. New studies demonstrate that women should be on a birth control pill with as *low* an estrogen level as possible to ensure fewer changes in the lipid factors.

I suggest that if you take oral contraceptives, they should be low in estrogen, with no more than 35 micrograms of this hormone per pill. Quite frankly, I am shocked that a doctor would continue to recommend a lifelong regimen of oral contraceptives. Kathy also has clear signs of premenstrual syndrome, possibly aggravated by the Pill. My advice to her or any woman taking oral contraceptives for endometriosis and suffering from PMS is to simply stop taking them now. Instead, I would advise a self-help, holistic regime, as noted in the previous chapter, emphasizing frequent small meals, an increase in B complex vitamins, avoidance of salt and sugar, and plenty of sleep and exercise.

If a laparoscopy has proved the presence of endometriosis and your symptoms are severe pain and cramping, and if your doctor prescribes birth control pills *as the first treatment of choice,* seek a second medical opinion elsewhere!

What Is Depo-Provera, and Can It Cure Endometriosis?

"I just turned thirty-six and I've been trying to get pregnant for ten years," wrote Patricia, a Louisiana real estate broker who is facing an infertility problem common to many women in their thirties. Patricia had a laparoscopy after complaints of chronic pain in her left side. The doctor found extensive endometriosis and an ovarian cyst. Her letter continued, "My doctor wants to treat me with something called Depo-Provera for at least one year. After the treatment, he thinks that I *may* have a chance of getting pregnant, but he cautioned that the effects of this hormone can delay conception for a long time after the treatment stops. I want to do the best thing, but without sacrificing time or my health, since I don't have too many fertile years left. A friend of mine took Depo-Provera and it cleared up her endometriosis, but she already had two children by that time and she didn't want any more. Will taking Depo-Provera do something to my hormones that could be irreversible?"

Depo-Provera is a synthetic progesterone that tends to elicit strong opinions from the medical establishment. Some doctors will not prescribe it and others see it as an excellent suppressant of the disease process of endometriosis. Depo-Provera, like the birth control pill given continuously, puts the body in a state of pseudopregnancy, creating a prolonged period of amenorrhea. The drug differs, though, in a number of unique ways.

A synthetic progesterone in an oil base, Depo-Provera is injected into muscle. Unlike oral contraceptives, which must be taken on a daily basis, this injected hormone is long-acting, and thus considered a convenience by both patients and doctors who favor it. The first injection may be effective from four weeks to two months, depending on the physician's program of using this drug. The subsequent shots can be given every six to ten weeks for one year, although some doctors continue the treatment "for as long as is necessary."

Put in a state of pseudopregnancy, a woman suffering from endometriosis is relieved of hormonal fluctuations and the concurrent problems associated with menstruation. Depo-Provera most often creates a state of amenorrhea, but there are chances of irregular though light bleeding patterns and spotting. Other side effects of the drug include pelvic pain, fatigue, headaches or migraines, and water retention.

It is important that women are informed of Depo-Provera's characteristically *long-term effects* before agreeing to this choice of treatment. Depo-Provera is not recommended for women who are interested in conceiving soon after treatment, since the most critical aftereffect of the drug is that it may not only suppress menstruation but may also *suppress ovulation for a year or more after the drug is discontinued*. That is how long it takes for the body to eliminate all traces of the drug. Taking fertility drugs to induce ovulation would not be the recommended course of action right on the heels of discontinuing Depo-Provera. This long-acting progestin will continue to block ovulation as long as it is potent in the body, even with the addition of fertility drugs.

Upjohn, the maker of Depo-Provera, has lobbied unsuccessfully to get it approved as a viable birth control drug. Unlike oral contraceptives, which still present the chance of worsening or causing cardiovascular problems to high-risk women, Depo-Provera tends not to cause such side effects because it does not contain estrogen. However, in a number of laboratory studies done on dogs, it was found to cause breast tumors.

In some cases where other medications such as Danocrine have been ineffective, Depo-Provera might work, if only to provide needed pelvic rest from menstruation. I have prescribed this hormone on a limited basis when a patient cannot tolerate Danocrine, which in my opinion is the more effective remedy for endometriosis. (More on this in a moment.) Again, Depo-Provera, like the oral contraceptive, will not shrink endometrial tissue. In fact, it may give areas of growth an appearance of being hemorrhagic, actually making surgery easier for doctors, since the tissue is more easily identified. The progesterone in the drug will keep the endometriosis tissue alive, and the disease will continue to spread when treatment is stopped.

For this reason, I would not recommend Depo-Provera to women like Patricia. If she is interested in having a child soon *after* treatment, my suggestion would be to take a different course. For example, a year's time may be necessary to shrink the endometriosis using a drug like Danocrine, taken in conjunction with the endometriosis diet and exercise. Depo-Provera should be used only in very select cases to keep endometriosis temporarily under control. This therapy would most likely involve patients who cannot tolerate any other medications given for the disease.

DO MALE HORMONES HELP TO STOP ENDOMETRIAL GROWTH?

Many women in the 1950s were given male hormones, or androgens, in low doses to stop menstrual cramping. Although there are other therapies of greater value, some doctors still hew to the old theory of using the male hormone testosterone as therapy for endometriosis.

"I wanted to end the pain, but I didn't want to become masculinized," one woman told me. "Male hormones left *irreversible* side effects. I can't get rid of superfluous body hair no matter what I do, and each month I have a bad acne outbreak." Her doctor had prescribed male hormones to control breakthrough bleeding, severe menstrual cramps, and painful intercourse. Now this woman is rightly concerned. In high doses, it has been shown that testosterone will decrease the effects of estrogen and progesterone, and thereby shrink endometrial lesions, but it is not a treatment of choice. There are often undesirable side effects, such as increase of body and facial hair and acne. Other effects of testosterone include increased musculature and a possible deepening of the voice.

A number of laboratory studies were conducted in the late 1970s using low-dosage androgens. Patients having endometriosis were put on male hormones for up to six months. Ovulation was not sup-

151

pressed, the endometrium showed no changes after treatment, but there was a cessation, in general, of symptomatic pain. If conception occurred while a woman was taking low-dosage androgens, a female child would have a greater chance of being born masculinized.

Since other drug therapies exist today that do not possess as many drawbacks, I would recommend that women veto any suggestion of a testosterone regimen to cure endometriosis or to reduce severe menstrual cramps.

CAN ESTROGEN HELP IN THE TREATMENT OF ENDOMETRIOSIS?

In the 1940s and 1950s, estrogen was prescribed for endometriosis in the form of Stilbestrol (DES). It was given to create the condition of amenorrhea and thus prevent the monthly retrograde flushing of tissue that could increase endometrial implants. Stilbestrol looked encouraging, as women tended to be helped by taking it. Many doctors were enthusiastic about such hormone therapy, and relied on Stilbestrol over other treatments, even surgical removal of endometrial lesions.

Continued experimentation, informed scrutiny, and laboratory analysis of this powerful hormone have proved that it must be given with wisdom and respect. In terms of helping women with endometriosis, no hormone could be more counterproductive. Endometrial tissue *proliferates* when it is fed estrogen. (In fact, studies indicate that women with naturally higher levels of estrogen are more likely to develop endometriosis.) Side effects of estrogen can be vaginal discharges, breakthrough (midmonth) bleeding, nausea, and breast tenderness. Most important, estrogen has been implicated in the growth of certain cancers and will also increase chances of thrombophlebitis, an inflammation of the wall of a vein, accompanied by formation of blood clots, most often occurring in the legs. If not diagnosed and treated, such a blood clot can travel through the circulatory system to the heart and lungs and be fatal.

Young women should avoid taking this hormone, since their own hormone levels tend to be high. Additional estrogen can be dangerous, causing breast cancer or heart attacks.

But what of women who are menopausal and who are on estrogen replacement therapy (ERT)? Menopause brings with it a lowering of estrogen and becomes, incidentally, one natural cure for endometriosis. Women who take estrogen replacement therapy to smooth the years-long transition from the reproductive years into complete menopause to end the uncomfortable symptoms of menopause—hot flashes, drying of vaginal walls, breast reduction, fatigue, weight gain, extreme mood swings—will find that the drug restimulates any inactive implants of endometriosis.

A menopausal woman should not be given estrogen replacement therapy to ease menopause until it can be ascertained that she is completely cured of her endometriosis. The woman herself is the first and best judge of this—she has lived with the disease and its symptoms for many years. If she is symptom-free for at least twelve months, and if her doctor examines her and finds no clinical signs of the disease (cysts or tumors), she may then be placed on this hormone.

Although individualized treatment must determine whether or not to give estrogen, I would not prescribe this hormone in the treatment of endometriosis.

DANOCRINE—THE FIRST TREATMENT OF CHOICE

Researchers looking for a drug therapy that would ease the symptoms of endometriosis 100 percent have come close in the use of danazol, or Danocrine (its brand name). This "antihormone" has become, in the last decade, the treatment of choice. Approved in 1976 by the FDA for the treatment of endometriosis, Danocrine has the benefit of shrinking endometrial tissue, suppressing ovarian production of hormones, and lessening the worst of menstruation-related symptoms.

Danocrine works on a simple principle. Since natural menopause is one natural cure for the disease, why not create this condition artificially? Without stimulation by the ovarian hormones, estrogen and progesterone, the endometrium shrinks, as do endometrial masses, and total healing is a long-term possibility. Danocrine is a gonadotropin inhibitor: it directly affects the FSH (follicle-stimulating hormone) and LH (luteinizing hormone) secretions of the hypothalamus and pituitary. These are the brain hormones that stimulate the production of ovarian hormones. As a result of Danocrine, ovulation is blocked, estrogen production is lowered, and the drug creates a pseudomenopause. Fortunately, the estrogen and progesterone levels rarely drop lower than they would following normal menstruation.

Danocrine has five basic functions:

1. As noted above, it directly affects the FSH and LH secretions of the hypothalamus and pituitary, thereby lowering estrogen production and blocking ovulation.

153

2. It blocks the estrogen and progesterone receptors in the endometrial cells so the tissue no longer is stimulated and actually begins to atrophy.

3. It inhibits secretion of the several enzymes that are involved in the production of estrogen and progesterone.

4. It alters the body's metabolism of estrogen and progesterone, by increasing the breakdown (or clearance) of these hormones. This metabolic alteration reduces the effect of hormones on endometrial implants so they cannot be stimulated to grow.

5. It is also possible that Danocrine fosters a sufferer's general improvement by strengthening the immune system. Just *how* Danocrine works through this system is not yet entirely clear. But it is an important consideration, since recent studies indicate that an altered immune response is a factor in onset of endometriosis.

How is Danocrine different from other hormones? Pseudopregnancy induced by birth control pills or progestins like Depo-Provera will reduce *symptoms* of endometriosis, such as pain, but these drugs will *not shrink* large masses or adhesions. Pseudopregnancy suppresses ovarian function, but the endometrial masses can actually soften, and this may worsen the condition. Danocrine, in contrast, will shrink endometrial implants and soften the tissue before it disintegrates. For thousands of women, it is the "miracle" cure. For others, it must be noted, the drug is barely tolerated, and not every woman is a candidate for treatment with it. (The illustration below shows how Danocrine blocks hormones at the ovarian level, resulting in a much more effective cure for endometriosis.)

Dosage: Danocrine and Diet

Danocrine is started on the first day of menstruation. When it was first given in 1971 during its testing stage, the recommended dose was 800 mg a day, divided into three doses. Duration of treatment was six to nine months, a period thought to be adequate time for the disease to regress. Dosage levels have been studied and compared, and some controversy still focuses on Danocrine's effectiveness in treating and curing infertility in patients with endometriosis.

In my own practice, I find the most successful program is to start a patient with 600 mg daily, divided into two doses. I suggest taking one tablet at night; three tablets at once is too strong a dose. A steady blood level of the hormone is better maintained when the system is not overloaded by one high dosage. The general aim is to keep a

EFFECT OF DANOCRINE

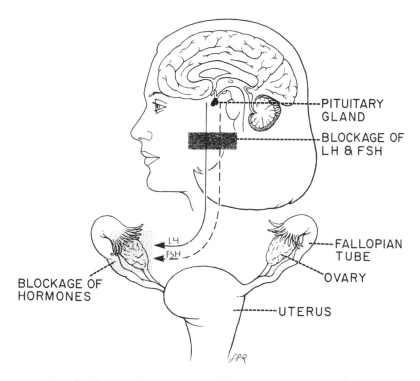

Used with permission of Winthrop Pharmaceuticals, New York, NY

patient on the drug until her condition improves, which is usually in six to nine months. Severe cases may require treatment for up to one year, while milder cases may need only five or six months. I usually find that the 600-mg dose can be maintained for the duration of treatment, although there are conditions where the dosage may need to be increased to 800 mg to stop midmonth or breakthrough bleeding, or (rarely) decreased to 400 mg daily. One problem commonly associated with dosage is irregular bleeding. Janice's case can help you understand what may happen.

Janice, who is twenty-eight years old, called me from North Carolina, where she was working as an assistant on film being shot on location. She had been taking Danocrine for three months. "I seem to be bleeding every few weeks," she told me, sounding worried. "Isn't Danocrine supposed to stop my period completely?"

Danocrine does stop menstruation, but the body is used to the estrogen-progesterone pattern of hormone fluctuation. It is common for women to have very light menstrual bleeding within the first three months of taking this medication. The body needs time to adjust to the hormonal levels that have been changed by Danocrine. After three months, breakthrough bleeding will usually disappear, although it might begin again after six or seven months on Danocrine. During the first month on Danocrine, a woman can expect a menstrual period that will be less painful, but perhaps longer than her normal period. The second period will be somewhat lighter and less painful, but can also last for several days—again, a few days more than is typical. The third period should be very much lighter or should not appear at all. This will vary from person to person. Women with fibroids or uterine abnormalities in addition to endometriosis (such as adenomyosis) often have bleeding that is more difficult to stop entirely.

If Janice is still bleeding into what would be her fourth menstrual period, I would want her to call me immediately. Then if I find that she is tolerating Danocrine without any adverse side effects (which I will talk about shortly), I would recommend her taking four tablets a day, or 800 mg. When the bleeding stops, the dose can be reduced again to 600 mg. If there is no cessation of bleeding by the fourth month, other measures must be taken. The next step might be progesterone tablets in the form of a 10-mg dose of Provera (not to be confused with Depo-Provera) once or twice daily with the Danocrine for five to ten days to see if the bleeding stops. The Provera helps to relax the uterus. An alternative progestin is Aygestin, which works like Provera. However, only a 5-mg dosage taken once or twice daily for the same amount of time is recommended for this drug. Doctors have also given Depo-Provera by injection. This drug is usually administered to women if they have been on Danocrine for three months and are still bleeding. Depo-Provera, remember, can remain in the body for up to a year or so, so it may be inadvisable if a woman is planning on pregnancy soon after the treatment.

If bleeding persists, and if blood tests are completely normal (for example, tests do not show kidney or liver dysfunction), I recommend 5 mg of vitamin K two or three times daily for a few weeks, since this vitamin enhances blood-clotting factors.

Most important, I never prescribe Danocrine without dietary advice. This drug should be supplemented by diet modification as well as by a vitamin program. Once on Danocrine, I advise women to increase their daily intake of vitamin C to 2,000 mg taken in four 500-mg doses along with a balanced 100-mg B complex tablet and 300–500 mg of B_6. I suggest small frequent meals and a reduction in sugar and salty foods. One very common side effect of the drug is water retention, which often requires that the woman also take a diuretic to cut down on bloating. Women can add approximately six to ten pounds of weight during the first three months of Danocrine therapy. After that, weight levels off and there is less bloating. Hormonal changes occurring in the body during pregnancy, due to birth control pills or Danocrine, all have an effect on the cells' retention of water. In pregnancy, the water retention creates a safer environment for the fetus, a sort of buffer system to protect it while also stabilizing body temperature. With Danocrine, there is an interaction between the drug and the adrenal glands and the kidneys, both of which regulate the rate of sodium excretion in the body.

There is really no rule to determine which woman will suffer from water retention due to Danocrine, although it has been found that women in warmer climates in general are more likely to retain water. This is probably related to a physiological adaptation to hot weather, where the body has learned to control water loss to guard against dehydration. Again, the tendency to edema depends on body build, nutritional status, and intake of salt in general.

If it is called for, I recommend a diuretic, or "water pill," such as Moduretic or Lasix, to be taken every other day if water retention is great and if edema is not improved by a salt-free diet. A unique type of drug, spironolactone, can not only be helpful as a diuretic but also has been found to have another beneficial effect: it will counteract the increase in body hair growth, one undesirable side effect of Danocrine, which affects a low percentage of women taking the drug. It can be taken in 25-mg doses once or twice a day for diuretic purposes and, if a woman's doctor feels it is necessary, in dosages from 100 to 200 mg a day to reduce hair growth.

(Spironolactone also has been used successfully with a high percentage of women who suffer from symptoms of PMS. Researchers have linked PMS to an oversupply of adrenal hormones, collectively called the aldosterone system. Spironolactone was found to relieve PMS symptoms and counteract fluid retention. This diuretic is recommended in its pure form, not in tablets containing spironolactone and hydrochlorothiazide, since the latter can contribute to a loss of body potassium. Any woman on hydrochlorothiazide requires monitoring.

157

It should be taken in low doses and in moderation, since laboratory studies have shown that high doses can cause malignancies in the breast and liver in animals. There have not been cases of such side effects in women, but nonetheless, it is wise to keep the dosage as low as possible.)

Aldactone (a brand name for the generic spironolactone)—25–200 mg daily—can also help reduce edema and is very helpful for women suffering from a variety of side effects of Danocrine. (See table of side effects, pages 160–161.)

Clarifying Three Myths About Danocrine

There are three important misconceptions about what Danocrine is and what it can do. Many women with endometriosis have heard of this drug, but hesitate to take it, fearing it will not help them as much as create further problems. Often this apprehension reflects a friend's experiences with unpleasant side effects from being on this antihormone. Most side effects are not serious and are short-term. My feeling is that if a doctor recommends this drug because he believes it will help his patient, a woman should give it a try.

These are the myths about the drug you are likely to hear:

Myth 1: Danocrine is a male hormone. This is not so. Danocrine inhibits ovarian production of estrogen, but the ovarian and adrenal androgens, the female body's own male hormones, are *not affected or suppressed* by the drug. With a lowered estrogen level, a woman's natural male hormone response is stronger.

Myth 2: This myth states that Danocrine creates the hormone levels found at menopause or following hysterectomy with removal of the ovaries. This is untrue. On Danocrine, a woman's estrogen level decreases to the level found right after menstruation, a time during the monthly cycle when many women feel better or at their best. Enough estrogen is always available to maintain other female functions.

Myth 3: This myth tells us that Danocrine is safe at any time. This is not the case. Before prescribing a drug like Danocrine, it must be determined that a woman is not pregnant. If she is pregnant or becomes pregnant (still a possibility) while on the drug, there is a slight chance of the drug causing genetic abnormality if the baby is a girl. Clitoral enlargement in girls is the only documented abnormality as a result of this drug so far; no genital abnormalities have been found among boys. Clearly, it is wise to use proper birth control measures to prevent conception while on the drug.

Monitoring the Effects of Danocrine

"How often must I be checked when I take this drug?"

"Which symptoms are normal and to be expected and which ones should I worry about?"

"How can I deal with side effects? I don't want to get discouraged and stop the drug too soon."

These are three questions I hear from patients every day when I start them on Danocrine. They are good questions—and perhaps critical to recovery. To get the most from Danocrine, you will need to be monitored carefully.

I prefer to see patients every six weeks during the entire course of treatment so I can judge how they are doing on it. I do a pelvic examination each time to determine if there is any decrease in the size of endometrial masses, put patients on the scale to see if there is any weight gain, in part due to edema, and take blood pressure. Every three months, women on Danocrine should have a blood test that includes liver profiles, evaluating the blood count, cholesterol level, and kidney function. There have been reports that Danocrine, like any other hormone such as birth control pills or fertility drugs, can affect liver function. Occasionally, there can be changes in the liver, which synthesizes hormones, creating some abnormality. Although this is extremely rare, normal liver function can be restored within a few weeks by stopping Danocrine. The liver is one of the faster-healing organs, regenerating quickly once the source of abnormality is found.

"How are you feeling?" It's a simple question, designed to find out if the patient has any symptoms or side effects. If there is a problem or two, we can make adjustments in the dosage, or design a different diet or vitamin regimen, or take her off the drug if she is unable to tolerate it. Side effects vary from woman to woman, and most will feel some change as the drug shifts the body into a state of pseudomenopause. I have heard women complain of little other than mild but persistent headaches and others complain of a wider range of discomfort. (I will discuss this in a moment.) It is also true that a great number of women report a renewed sense of well-being, since the drug has eliminated pelvic pain and PMS symptoms.

Managing Side Effects of Danocrine

Many studies have followed patients on Danocrine from the first innovative report by Georgia gynecologist Robert Greenblatt, M.D.,

POSSIBLE SIDE EFFECTS OF DANOCRINE

Side Effect	Management
Weight gain	Reduce salt intake
Fatigue or weakness	Modify diet
Dizziness	Mild diuretic such as spironolactone
Headaches	Avoid sugar, eat frequent small meals
	Increase intake of B complex to 100 mg; B_6 to 500 mg
	Use prostaglandin inhibitors such as Motrin
Acne	Antibiotics a possible treatment
Mild hirsutism	Spironolactone
Increased oiliness of skin and scalp	Reduce dose of Danocrine
Bleeding	Increase dosage if possible
Spotting	Progesterone tablets or Depo-Provera injections
Pelvic pain	Increase calcium and magnesium
Back pain	Decrease salt
	Lift properly
	Use prostaglandin inhibitors
Vaginitis	Specific treatment if infection is found
	Douche with Betadine
	Antiyeast cream and suppositories
	Reduce sugar intake
Decrease in breast size	Breast size will return to normal when treatment is terminated
Breast tenderness and swelling	Diuretics
Localized breast pain and/ or painful lumps that do not decrease in size	Evaluate for cancer

Side Effect	Management
Muscle cramps Back and neck aches	Mild diuretics if necessary Reduce salt intake Increase calcium and magnesium Low-salt, high-calcium diet

Hot flashes, flushes,
   sweating
	Reduce dosage of Danocrine
	B-complex, B_6, calcium, magnesium,
	   vitamin E

Depression, sleeplessness,
   anxiety
	Diet modification, increase vitamin
	   intake
	Spironolactone
	Mild sleeping pills
	Tryptophan
	Reduce dosage

Rash
Increased allergies
	Investigate cause
	Treatment with cortisone creams or
	   other topical medication
	Antihistamines such as Benadryl or
	   Chlor-Trimiton

Adapted from Danazol Side Effects/Summary and Management, *Managing Danazol Patients,* © Creative Informatics, Inc.

and his colleagues in 1971, five years before the drug was officially approved as a treatment for endometriosis. At that time, as I have mentioned, dosage was initiated at 800 mg a day, which was considered the amount needed to produce shrinkage of endometrial masses. But many women suffered unpleasant side effects at this dosage.

In one more recent multipurpose comparative study led by Dr. Veasy Buttram at the Baylor College of Medicine, the team compared an 800-mg regimen with a 400-mg regimen with regard to side effects, resolution of the disease, and enhancement of conception rates. Of 220 patients participating in the study, 7 percent discontinued medication primarily because of depression and muscle cramping, and did not continue the six-month course of medication. In fact, there were twice the number of side effects that necessitated discontinuation of the drug among those taking the higher dose than the lower. Weight gain, an aforementioned side effect, was present in 85 percent of the patients, but the weight was pretty much kept to under ten pounds (although 41 percent of women taking 800 mg a day gained more weight than those receiving 400 mg).

Over the twelve years since danazol's acceptance as the preferred medical approach, doctors and researchers have found that the positive effects of Danocrine far outweigh the side effects. What can be expected, then, from Danocrine?

"I've been on 800 mg of Danocrine for a month," wrote Joan, a twenty-seven-year-old publicist from Chicago, "and by the end of the second week, I felt awful. I started spotting, had headaches on and off all day, and gained seven pounds. By the third week, I had a bloody-looking spot inside my mouth. Then came the skin rash and some hair loss. By the end of the fourth week I had to stop. I still have pain from endometriosis as before. What can I do?"

This note to me describes what *may* happen on a dosage this high. Weight gain because of fluid retention, as previously mentioned, is a symptom common to hormone supplementation. However, Joan's other symptoms can be reduced or eliminated by changing the dosage to 600 mg a day. If there are still problems, the dosage should again be reduced to 400 mg. You also need to remember that irritability, nervousness, and some pain are expected in the beginning of any new hormone regimen. Like Joan, you might not feel very well until you adjust to the new level of hormones. The body is very sensitive to hormone changes and I urge women to give the drug a chance, taking care to watch salt and sugar intake, increase vitamin intake, and use diuretics wisely.

Other Side Effects of Danocrine

Acne: Your doctor might put you on antibiotics, such as tetracycline or another anti-acne medication such as Accutane, if the skin condition is exceptionally bad. If acne persists, a lowered dosage of Danocrine may help.

Vaginal infections: Because of lowered estrogen levels, some women taking Danocrine might get monilia, a yeast infection. I suggest they avoid sugar and fermented products, which promote such infections. It is also advisable not to wear panty hose or tight synthetic fabric underpants or pants. Treatment: douche with a povidine-iodine solution, such as Betadine, at bedtime. If a doctor advises it, use a vaginal suppository to help clear up the infection.

Breast reduction: The decline in estrogen levels may cause the breasts to decrease in size. If you suffer from fibrocystic disease, Danocrine might be of special help, since it also shrinks these cysts in the breast. In fact, the FDA has approved this drug for the treatment of this common breast disorder. It has been thought that on a regimen of Danocrine for six to nine months, women with fibrocystic disease are at less risk for breast cancer, since hormones are kept at a steady level. Breast size usually returns to normal within two months following the completion of drug therapy.

Leg cramps: A number of women complain of leg cramping. This could be due to some water retention in the muscles, which irritates the nerves, or it could be the effect of a low calcium level. I would recommend working with your doctor to devise a program of calcium supplements, mild diuretics, and a low-salt diet.

Androgenic effects: Some women will experience side effects that appear to be masculinizing, such as a slight increase in growth of body and facial hair (hirsutism), a slight deepening of the voice, and oilier skin. These effects are clearly traced to a decline in natural estrogen levels while on Danocrine, but they do not occur in every case.

Side effects vary from individual to individual. The table below shows the known side effects that may appear, and how they can be managed.

THE NEW GnRH ANALOGS

"I had a bad reaction to Danocrine, and my endometriosis is too advanced for me to take the birth control pill. Is there any drug that can help me?"

I am often asked this question by women who have not had the best of experiences with Danocrine or other hormone treatments. Over the last few years, research has been intensified to find improved methods of treating and curing endometriosis. Right now, Danocrine is the closest *approved* medication, but a new breed of hormone "analogs" are being developed which look promising.

These analogs are called gonadotropin–releasing hormone analogs, or GnRH (or LH/RH) analogs. As of this writing, GnRH analogs are in the experimental stage and are not approved by the FDA. But the testing continues to uncover their range of capabilities. Powerful drugs, analogs have been used not only to shrink uterine fibroids but also to help endometriosis sufferers in a number of ways.

163

However, there are a few side effects inherent in them that can be counterproductive.

How Do Analogs Work?

To understand how analogs work, we need to review a basic fact about endometriosis: ovarian involvement. A decrease in estrogen levels—achieved either by removal of the ovaries (oophorectomy) or by suppression of ovarian functions with drugs—has been observed as an effective medical treatment of endometriosis. Of the two, the less drastic measure is drug-induced ovarian manipulation, where estrogen levels can be controlled. In this case, estrogen output is suppressed to a level that renders it incapable of stimulating endometriosis growth.

Danocrine (danazol) is one such avenue used to control estrogen; GnRH analogs, or agonists, are others. Both medications share a critical function: danazol and the agonists inhibit the hypothalamus-pituitary-ovarian functions. The hypothalamus produces FSH (follicle-stimulating hormone) and LH (luteinizing hormone) and stores them in the pituitary. A GnRH analog will *inhibit* the pituitary from secreting these hormones, which would signal the ovaries to produce estrogen and progesterone. Thus do agonists suppress ovarian function. Danazol and the agonists both *suppress hormone secretion* and *shrink* existing endometrial masses. Danazol may produce androgenlike side effects, however, while the gonadotropin-releasing hormones do not. Agonists have been shown to cause high calcium excretion (which can cause osteoporosis, or thinning of the bones), while danazol does not. Agonists of GnRH do not interact directly with receptors in endometrial tissue, but danazol has this desirable quality, which is why it is so effective. How feasible, then, are agonists (or antagonists, as they are also called) as long-term treatments for endometriosis?

The agonists backed into the world of endometriosis treatments; their origins were in a different but related field. At first, experiments were being done to search for a safer, more effective birth control pill. Oral contraceptives, composed of estrogen and progesterone, fool the brain and the body into thinking it is already pregnant, so that conception will not occur. Agonists, however, establish pseudomenopause, as does the related "antihormone," danazol. When FSH and LH do not stimulate the ovaries, the ovaries do not produce estrogen and progesterone, and so the body is in a pseudomenopausal state. The problem with using agonists for birth control was the unpleasant and immediate side effects—wide mood swings, hot flashes, backaches, headaches, and a greater risk of osteoporosis. This, then, was not the ideal formula for contraceptive use, since birth control pills are used over a long period of time, increasing the danger of calcium depletion.

Instead, the agonists *appeared* to be an effective alternative to danazol. Thus, by creating a reversible "medical oophorectomy" with the GnRH analogs, researchers hoped to find an answer to endometriosis. However, with all the adverse side effects, these agonists are not ready for widespread use in treating endometriosis.

How Agonists Can Help in the Fight to Cure Endometriosis

Unlike danazol, which is taken in tablet form, the GnRH agonists are destroyed by stomach acids and therefore cannot be ingested. Researchers have found two alternate routes of supplying the body with full-strength agonists: by nasal spray (intranasally) and by injection. One such GnRH agonist, called Buserelin, given both by injection and intranasally, was tested extensively in Quebec, Canada, by Dr. André LeMay, a specialist in endocrinology and reproductive medicine, and his colleagues. Nine women with severe endometriosis were treated with Buserelin for twenty-five to thirty-one weeks, and results looked promising. There was an immediate reduction in pain. Endometrial implants shrank and ovulation returned, on the average, forty-five days after the treatment was stopped (in fact, two women became pregnant within that time period). Side effects were typical of menopausal symptoms, such as vaginal dryness and hot flashes. Other studies focusing on Buserelin in treating endometriosis indicated improvement among most women who participated.

Led by Dr. K. A. Steingold, a team of doctors at the University of California's Division of Reproductive Endocrinology, Department of Obstretics and Gynecology, treated sixteen volunteers with endometriosis. Their conclusions were similar to the Quebec team's: there was marked relief in pelvic pain and suppression of the disease, but there were accompanying menopausal levels of calcium excretion. Many women also had insomnia and emotional disturbances and some experienced vaginal dryness. Two patients in the test were found to be free of endometriosis, but for others, the disease was not eradicated. In a third investigation using nafarelin, an agonist administered via nasal spray, early studies indicated that most women improved after only three months on the drug.

Agonists appear to be a likely alternative to Danocrine, but there are still some problems associated with them. Uppermost is the calcium loss caused by the drug, and severe hot flashes. Recent experiments with the agonists involve their use along with high-dosage calcium supplements. So far, it has been proved that 1,500 mg of this mineral can help offset the loss caused by the drug. However, some side effects once apparent are not reversible, and osteoporosis is one that might severely limit the use of this drug.

Others in the field are attempting to find a balanced formula of hormones that would counteract the menopausal side effects of the analogs without reducing their overall effectiveness in controlling endometriosis. Some scientists have begun their search by looking to the long-acting progestins such as Depo-Provera for use in combination with these potent GnRH drugs. So far, experiments have shown that injectible Depo-Provera tends to keep endometriotic tissue active, reducing the effect of the analog taken with it.

As of the publication of this book, GnRH agonists have not been approved for use in treating endometriosis. Agonists have great potential in treating the disease, but several researchers have not found them as effective as Danocrine. Once approved by the FDA, agonists may well offer an alternative treatment for select patients who cannot take Danocrine.

WHAT HORMONE TREATMENT SHOULD YOU CHOOSE?

Each woman's case must be evaluated on its own terms. Individualized treatment is the only safe solution. You might be suffering from severe pain, but it's possible that a small dosage of Danocrine—two tablets twice a day—for just a few months will be enough to relieve symptoms and melt away the disease. It is realistic, in some cases, to rely on exercise and nutritional therapy, as noted earlier in this book. Again, it may be birth control pills that will help at early stages of endometriosis. Your options for improvement and cure may lie in a combination of drugs and dietary factors.

The information in this chapter should increase the understanding of your specific problem and help to guide you in considering various treatments. But it is your doctor who will need to determine, finally, what is right for you. If, after a program of treatment, you are not feeling better or are totally confused by your doctor's advice, remember, you have a choice: get another opinion from a physician who cares about your well-being.

CHAPTER 11

Lasers: The Most Successful Surgical Technique for Endometriosis

$\mathbf{M}$ENTION the word "lasers," and images of *Star Wars* weaponry and Jedi warriors come to mind. The laser "gun" in this highly popular film harnessed a vibrating beam of colored light that wielded a ferocious power: what it touched simply vanished without a trace. The *surgical* laser, the newest tool in the battle against endometriotic lesions, has been mistakenly regarded as such a force. It is a popular notion that a surgeon need only point the laser to "zap" the disease, cleanly, bloodlessly, and without any need for abdominal incisions.

This touch-and-zap surgical procedure does not exist, and could never be developed for treating endometriosis. Nor does such futuristic imagery capture the delicacy, precision, and versatility of the instrument or the kind of knowledge and skill that is required of the operating doctor. Laser surgery is a relatively new technique, astonishing in some ways and limited in others. For the woman with endometriosis, it may be one way to eradicate *some* of the disease, especially when it is used in tandem with specific medication (if it is indicated) and a concentrated effort to change diet and life-style.

Laser surgery was an inevitability as a surgical tool. As the number of women who suffer from endometriosis continues to rise, more research is being done by a larger group of scientists throughout the world to refine different treatment options. Laser and its newest innovation, videolaseroscopy, or the use of video monitoring devices with zoom lenses that magnify the areas that will be treated, are revolutionizing surgical procedures in the care and cure of endometriosis.

Laser, though an excellent tool in the hands of a good surgeon, is not for every woman with endometriosis. Remember, it is *surgery* wherein (in the case of a laparotomy) an abdominal incision will be made (to insert a laparoscope) *before* any laser surgery can begin. It may be able to create miracles for some, and certainly provide relief for many, but it will not work for everyone. Knowing where you fit on this spectrum is essential to undertaking treatment wisely.

How Is Laser Different from Other Forms of Surgery?

"I read in *Newsweek* about laser surgery removing endometriosis, but my doctor thought it would not help my case," wrote Judith, a thirty-three-year-old grade school teacher from Ohio. Her letter was one of many I received from women who did not know what laser could do for them. Judith continued, "I went to five other gynecologists and they all voted it down, too. One told me that lasers were dangerous and burn right through organs. My original doctor says that standard surgery will clean up my endometriosis. I had appendicitis, peritonitis, and a dermoid cyst removed, all between the ages of seventeen and eighteen. The operations left me with severe adhesions, especially around my uterus. A laparoscopy showed a lot of endometriosis on my tubes. I would not like to go through abdominal surgery again, but I have been unable to get pregnant after ten years of trying. Why wouldn't laser be preferable to 'going under the knife'? Why would six doctors discourage its use in my case?"

The article to which Judith referred brought laser techniques greater public recognition for battling, as *Newsweek* called it, "the career woman's disease." Laser surgery suddenly seemed to bring a promise of hope to many sufferers of endometriosis. Many hopeful women, like Judith, are attracted to laser's many advantages. One is minimal blood loss (which cuts down on the need for transfusions). Others are that surgery may take far less time than conventional surgery and require a shorter recovery period.

"Used properly, laser is the best surgical tool known to man for the eradication of endometriotic tissue," says Dr. J. Victor Reyniak, a clinical professor of gynecology and obstetrics and director of reproductive endocrinology at the Mount Sinai School of Medicine in New York City. A highly reputed specialist in laser surgery for this condition, Dr. Reyniak posed a comparison: "There are three basic surgical methods to diminish endometriosis. You can apply *kinetic* energy, that is, surgery can be done entirely with a surgical knife. But not all cases of endometriosis justify exposing the abdomen to laparotomy, or major surgery. Next, you can apply *electrical* energy, or cautery. With cauterization an electrical current devitalizes the tissue and causes tissue sloughing, but it might invite the formation of adhesions." Cautery is also limited, since it is a process wherein organs can be burned unless it is used carefully and skillfully.

"Finally," he continued, "you can apply *light* energy, as with a laser. With laser, you can remove endometriotic lesions layer by layer with ultimate precision. The laser doesn't leave any residue, but it does leave a clean crater of laser impact. Under these conditions, the area doesn't invite other organs to stick to it and develop adhesions, since only minute incisions are made through the laparoscope.

"Which sounds less traumatic? I believe it is the laser, a true twenty-first-century surgical tool."

Why does laser provide all these advantages? Let's see how the instrument operates.

How Lasers Work

The laser is often used along with the laparoscope, thereby making extensive abdominal surgery unnecessary. The laparoscopy is performed in the usual way with a half-inch incision made in the navel, in which the laparoscope is inserted. The surgeon inserts the laser through the operating channel of the instrument. A second tiny incision is made above the pubic bone and a probe inserted. This probe suctions out the rinsing solutions and debris from the lasered tissue. When it is necessary, a third tiny incision is made for grasping tools, which manipulate or move internal organs. In videolaseroscopy, a miniature video camera with a zoom lens is mounted on the laparoscope. The surgeon operates with the laser by looking at the screen, where tissue can be magnified up to twenty times its size.

Surgery using the video may appear to be difficult, dangerous, or slightly haphazard. But this is not so. Before videolaseroscopy, simple laser laparoscopies were a greater strain for physicians. Dr. Camran Nezhat, a gynecologist associated with the Fertility and Endocrinology Center in Atlanta and one of the prime innovators of this technique, reported on this procedure in an issue of *Obstetrics and Gynecology Forum*. In comparing the disadvantages of the earlier procedure, he stated that since the laparoscope allows the use of only one eye peering through a narrow aperture, "the physician's field of view is limited and poor visualization of the peritoneal structure and pathology may result. . . . Videolaseroscopy allows the surgeon to operate in an upright position directly from the videomonitor, reducing back strain and fatigue." Normally, the doctor must constantly bend over the patient's abdomen to see through the laparoscope. With the camera, the surgeon operates using both eyes. He can also magnify the ovaries and tubes and zoom in on areas of endometriosis, no matter how deep in the pelvis the implants may be.

The laser instruments are simple-looking tools fueled by common gases; they are the argon laser and the carbon dioxide laser (the latter is familiarly called the CO_2 laser). The argon laser does not "cut" or vaporize tissue, but it will cause blood coagulation to stop bleeding. The argon laser is also attracted to red dye, and therefore, areas with a lot of blood, such as areas inflamed by endometrial implants, will be most affected by it. Argon travels along a flexible fiber, which is one of its distinctive qualities. The CO_2 laser only works in a direct straight line. If the surgeon is confronted by a large endometriotic cyst, and he finds it difficult to work with the CO_2 laser because it will not turn a corner, he may switch to the argon flexible fiber to get around the corner and vaporize the tissue within the confines of the cyst.

The CO_2 laser is actually a molecular gas laser which emits an intense and "coherent" beam of infrared light that is focused on, but is not directly touching, its target. Rather, the beam of light is pointed at the tissue, while the instrument is held a few centimeters above it. The laser's reputation as the "touch-and-zap" tool stems from the actual surgical process, sometimes called vaporization.

The wavelength of the laser's infrared beam tends to be absorbed by water. Human body cells are mostly water. When the laser is applied to soft tissue, like an endometriotic lesion, the water in the cells begins to heat rapidly, or, as it has been aptly described, "flash-boil." The heated water follows its nature and is converted to steam. The surgeon can almost observe a small explosion as the steam expands or explodes the cells that have been irradiated by the laser. What remains is cell debris, and the telltale "laser plume," the smoke from the vaporization of the tissue. The end result is that the diseased cells are totally destroyed, including their DNA, so that if a fragment were to remain, it could not reproduce itself.

The laser can be adjusted to provide ultimate precision for vaporizing minute areas. The size of the beam of light can be made as small as .2 millimeters, and the depth of penetration of a single laser burst can be 500 microns, or half a millimeter, in depth. Such microsurgery allows the doctor to vaporize cell layers one at a time. For larger masses, a doctor can excise and lift endometriotic lesions off vital organs, like the bowel or the bladder, without damaging them, by vaporizing cell layers surrounding and underlying the structure. (See illustration. Note that the laser beam, reflected in the small mirror, is pointed toward the endometrial implant, and the implant is subsequently vaporized and destroyed.)

Vaporization has a number of other special benefits:

• Laser is "cleaner" surgery. The heat of vaporization cuts down on bleeding from the smaller blood vessels like capillaries, and the vaporized tissue can be quickly siphoned out. In cases of extreme uterine

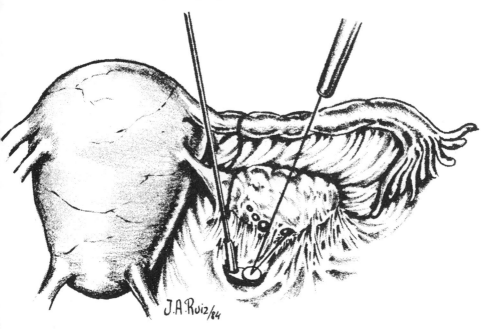

Vaporization of endometriosis using the reflecting power of the laser.

Used with permission of Michael S. Baggish, M.D., editor, *Basic and Advanced Laser Surgery in Gynecology,* Appleton-Century-Crofts

bleeding, laser has been used to selectively destroy the abnormal tissues lining the uterus. Severe and uncontrolled uterine bleeding was once treated by hysterectomy, but with laser, the uterus is left intact and the recovery rate is much faster. (This particular procedure is not recommended for women who still want to have children, since it causes sterilization.)

• Adhesions, which are fibrous bands of tissue that may grow and abnormally connect the surfaces of organs, can be very carefully vaporized, even along the hair-thin fallopian tubes. To do this, the surgeon will insert other instruments to lift the tubes or move organs for better viewing and remove the adhesions cell layer by cell layer. Laser laparoscopy is known to prevent the development of new adhesions. When the peritoneal cavity is exposed to air, as in conventional surgery, it begins to dry under operating room lights and can invite adhesions.

• Since the abdomen is not opened, risk of infection is greatly reduced. With laser laparoscopy, only the sterilizing laser beam touches the diseased tissue—there is no handling of other organs by doctors or sterilized instruments.

• Postoperative recovery rates are usually excellent. On the average, patients can be discharged from the hospital four *hours* later. Side effects and complications, so far, are no more extensive than gas pains and slight bruising of the abdominal wall from the laparoscope.

• The CO_2 laser, in particular, can be especially helpful for women who do not have large endometriotic cysts and are looking for relief from pain—all accomplished through a tiny incision in the navel. Bigger cysts may call for laparotomy, but the surgeon could still use a combination of scalpel and lasers during this abdominal surgery. Depending on the case, he may choose to cut away larger cysts or tumors using the scalpel, then switch to the laser to eradicate other endometrial implants.

CAN LASER SURGERY END SEVERE MENSTRUAL CRAMPS?

A patient recently diagnosed as having endometriosis called me to ask about surgery to reduce her pain. Sarah, who is twenty-three years old and working as a computer programmer, has, in the past, been incapacitated a few days a month by endometriosis pain. She has started on Danocrine treatment, along with a change of diet, but she fears that when she goes off the medication, nutritional changes will not be enough to keep her pain-free. Sarah thinks that since she has endometriosis now, she will always have it, and that it is just a matter of time before it grows back.

She told me, "I heard from a friend that a few doctors at the Wayne State College of Medicine are using laser surgery to cut the ligaments behind the uterus to stop pain from endometriosis. How can cutting these ligaments stop menstrual cramps? If I have this surgery, will it interfere with my having a baby in the future?"

Nerve tissue to the uterus stems from the uterosacral ligament, which is found behind this organ. For a long time it was felt that menstrual pain could be reduced by cutting and shortening the uterosacral ligament, thereby changing the position of the uterus, or "suspending" it. (One result of endometriotic growths is that they can pull the uterus backward, out of position. "Suspending" it pulls it forward to its normal position.)

CAN LASER SURGERY HELP YOU?

Laser techniques work best for

(1) women who have moderate to severe cases of endometriosis and clearly visible endometrial cysts or masses, and who have not responded to drug treatments and (2) women with adhesions on the bladder, uterus, fallopian tubes, and ovaries. (A surgeon may do lysis, a freeing of adhesions from abdominal and pelvic organs, using laser laparoscopy. However, there may be more severe cases where it is necessary to have exploratory surgery to remove adhesions behind the uterus with a scalpel.)

Laser surgery cannot help women with mild endometriosis who do not have visible lesions. Laser can only vaporize the endometriosis that the doctor can see. When there are microscopic implants, the organs just look inflamed. It is impossible to aim a laser at any one of millions of spots and hope it is an implant. (To get an idea of the difficulty of such a task, rub your hands together vigorously, then look at your palms. They are rosy from increased circulation to the area. Now imagine trying to vaporize away the rosiness, spot by spot.)

WHAT TO DO BEFORE AND AFTER
LASER SURGERY

If you have not responded to drug treatments and your doctor feels that you are a candidate for laser surgery, try to get yourself in as good a condition as you can before entering the hospital. You want to strengthen your immune system. My recommendations follow, but be sure to check with your doctor before using any of these guidelines:

BEFORE LASER SURGERY:
• *Watch your diet.* Cut down on fats, salt, and sugary food. Increase your daily intake of complex carbohydrates (whole-grain foods) and vegetables. These foods are not only nutritionally sound but help to cleanse the bowel.
• *Increase vitamins.* For at least a week prior to surgery, take vitamins on a daily basis that strengthen immune systems. They are beta-carotene (10,000 IU), vitamin B_6 (500 mg), B complex (one balanced-formula tablet), vitamin C (1,500 mg, divided into three doses of 500 mg), vitamin E (800 IU a day, divided into two doses of 400 IU), and zinc (50 mg).
• *Take mild exercise.* Exercise benefits your cardiovascular system as well as your mood. Strenuous exercise should be ruled out, but walking at an easy pace about fifteen minutes to half an hour a day can help.
• *Maintain a positive attitude.* It is natural to be apprehensive about going in for any type of surgery, but do not dwell on any unpleasant thoughts. This adds unnecessary stress. Be kind to yourself and try to remain calm.

AFTER LASER SURGERY:
• *Have someone waiting to take you home.* Most women can leave the hospital from four to twelve hours following laser surgery. Since the procedure is done under anesthesia, you will need to have a relative or friend with you when you check out of the hospital. Most women feel perfectly fine after the anesthetic wears off, but some may be slightly nauseated or even a bit dizzy.
• *Give yourself a chance to recover.* Even if you feel good

the day after surgery, do not get right back into a hectic schedule. Allow at least two weeks for proper healing. Don't overload on activities.

• *Continue on the presurgery vitamin plan.* Take the same doses of beta-carotene, vitamins B_6, B complex, C, and E, and zinc as noted above for at least two weeks postoperatively.

• *Follow the endometriosis diet.* What you eat now will influence your health and well-being way into the future. If you have had laser surgery to vaporize endometriosis, you have a chance to help prevent recurrence of the disease by watching your diet.

• *Follow up treatment with medications.* Your doctor will be able to determine if you require any drug treatments, such as Danocrine, following surgery. You may be asked to take Danocrine for three to six months to shrink any implants that are microscopic.

The Wayne State team conducted studies on about sixty patients with uncontrollable menstrual cramps. They used a combination of laser laparoscopy and electrocautery to vaporize the uterosacral ligament. Their conclusion was that pain is greatly reduced in most cases. Several other physicians are using this double procedure and are satisfied with the results. My thinking is that menstrual cramping may be *somewhat* reduced by such surgery, but I would not recommend it as the first treatment of choice, since it does not relieve pain for every patient. If Sarah chooses to have this surgery, it will not interfere with her bearing a child in the future.

Will Sarah's endometriosis recur, even if such surgery is performed on her? Dr. Veasy C. Buttram, a leading authority on endometriosis, has reported on its recurrence rate. He found that the single most important factor in endometriosis recurrence is the ovary. If the ovaries are involved, over 90 percent of cases will recur; if the ovary is not involved, 47 percent of women will experience a recurrence within ten years of treatment. Can laser help to reduce recurrence?

Dr. J. Victor Reyniak, introduced earlier, says, "Since the laser vaporizes the DNA of the cell, it appears logical that the recurrence rate will be lower, but we don't know yet. Laser surgery is still too new and our follow-up is insufficient to judge that. I feel hopeful that laser will make a difference."

How Important Is Laser for Curing Infertility?

Laser laparoscopy has changed the course of many women's lives who were previously unable to have children when endometriosis was implicated. Prostaglandins produced by endometriotic tissue can interfere with ovulation and the release of eggs. Laser surgery in this case could be helpful. However, if tubes are not patent, or open, because endometriotic growths have obstructed them, chances for conception are severely diminished even after laser treatment.

"If I have laser surgery, can I have a baby?" Women with infertility problems related to endometriosis place much hope on this surgery. Although surgeons would like to guarantee a 100 percent chance of conception, this is impossible. There are instances when endometriosis is only one factor in causing infertility. Others are complications involving the chemistry of cervical mucus, the condition of the fallopian tubes, the man's sperm count and sperm motility, and any number of known or unknown issues.

It is my feeling that laser surgery can be used effectively in combination with other treatments and a change in diet for the woman with more extensive endometriosis who *does not want to conceive right away*. She could undergo laser surgery to vaporize visible lesions and then begin a program of Danocrine treatment to help eliminate any microscopic growths. After four to six months on Danocrine, I would recommend a low-dosage oral contraceptive, such as Nordette, Ortho-Novum 1/35, Tri-Norinyl, Loestrin Fe 1.5/30, Demulen 1/35, Levlen, Ovcon 35, or any modification of these birth control pills as tolerated by each woman.

With this combination of therapies, over a year's time, the body should heal itself and the endometriosis disappear.

What about the woman who does want to conceive immediately after laser surgery? If her recovery is successful and if she finds she is not pregnant within a year of the surgery, only a thorough workup with a fertility expert can answer her questions. Dr. Camran Nezhat of Atlanta performs videolaseroscopy frequently. He has found that of 631 patients in his study, 441 agreed to surgery because of infertility problems. Of these women, 181 had at least one other factor that contributed to not conceiving.

Looking closer at his study, 260 patients had endometriosis as the single factor blocking conception. Of them, Dr. Nezhat and his colleagues followed 156 women postoperatively. Their study shows promise: 65 percent became pregnant within eighteen months, the greater proportion conceiving within six months of surgery.

In my own studies involving postlaser surgery follow-ups among women with endometriosis, I have found that the chances of conception are even higher. However, conception often requires aggressive treatment with fertility drugs. In some cases, artificial insemination may be the answer. Women who have not conceived using these techniques might also be excellent candidates for *in vitro* fertilization, which will be described in the next chapter.

FINDING THE RIGHT DOCTOR TO PERFORM LASER SURGERY

More doctors than ever are using the CO_2 and argon lasers. *But not every doctor can do it effectively and safely.* The nature of laser technology demands expertise. Defocused laser beams under certain circumstances can cause cauterization, or burning, instead of vaporization of tissue.

Doctors must be trained in laser procedures and gain experience with them, as is true with any surgical technique. How, then, would you know if *your* doctor can work competently with the laser? If he is doing the surgery himself, you will have to ask him a number of questions before agreeing to it. If he recommends laser surgery and refers you to another doctor who he believes is a specialist, you still will need to ask these questions:

- Why do you think I would benefit from laser surgery?
- Where did you learn how to use the laser?
- Have you trained intensively with a known expert in the field? If so, who is he and at what medical center does he train others?
- Was your training focused on abdominal and pelvic laser laparoscopy?
- How many laser laparoscopies for endometriosis do you estimate you have done in the last year?
- Do you know how I might contact a woman who has had successful laser surgery for this condition? I would like to speak to her because it will help me to understand this procedure from the patient's point of view.
- Do you attend seminars or lectures on the most up-to-date laser techniques?
- How much will it cost?

You should be aware that laser is very expensive and few doctors own such equipment privately. It is more often found in medical centers and hospitals, where many doctors have access to it, and the cost of surgery may reflect this. A few obstetrical and gynecological journals report that some doctors charge more for laser surgery, justifying the cost by citing the special training that is required of them—and perhaps even "overselling" the procedure. This is another reason why it is wise to get a second opinion before submitting to it.

Finally, you might also contact the American Society for Laser Medicine and Surgery (see appendix) for further information about the technique and how to judge your doctor's experience and expertise with it.

Although laser surgery has made great impact in treating cases of endometriosis, I must emphasize that *it is not for every woman with this condition*. Early stages of endometriosis might be cured or alleviated by diet, vitamins, and hormone treatments alone. Other cases could need medical treatment with Danocrine or the newer and soon-to-be-available agonists mentioned in the previous chapter. Remember that your case is unique. Laser surgery is a formidable option, but use it wisely!

CHAPTER 12

Infertility and Endometriosis: You Can Have a Baby

HAVING a baby can be one of the most important events in a woman's life. It is a time when many women feel emotionally and physically "complete" as they go through the miraculous process of bearing a child. Others find a natural, easy comfort in creating a family life, but are not so easy about the state of pregnancy itself. There are also women who do not want children, but who are content to know that they *could* get pregnant if they so chose. If biology is destiny, then those women who want children and bear them have no argument with nature. But what happens when biology is skewed by endometriosis that changes—or delays—a woman's preferred destiny to have a child?

In my experience, I have found that there are many variations of what may happen to prevent conception when endometriosis is present. Physical or hormonal aberrations or a combination of the two may render a woman infertile. Many women who cannot conceive, in spite of no apparent abnormalities, are now referred to as having "unexplained infertility." In some cases, I believe their problem is caused by undiagnosed endometriosis.

Surgery, medications, fertility drugs, artificial insemination, and *in vitro* fertilization open a wide range of possibilities for the temporarily infertile woman. If you really want a baby, there is hope for you! Studies have shown that women with endometriosis have twice the fertility problems as those who are free of the disease. This is a fact of life right now, but with good medical care, some of these statistics may be reversed. It was recently reported in *OB.GYN News* that first-year pregnancy rates after danazol therapy for infertility due to endometriosis were 37 percent for women with severe cases, 72 percent with moderate disease symptoms, and 83 percent for those with mild cases. This is good news! After treatment with medications *and* conventional surgery or laser laparoscopy, other studies show, more than half of women are able to conceive. Such statistics are extremely promising.

"I was pregnant twice, but I wasn't ready for motherhood," a new patient told me. "So I had an abortion each time. Ten years later, I can't get pregnant now that I want to. I know I ovulate. I can feel it every month, so the endometriosis can't be *too* severe. What can be done to help me?" Another patient told me, "I did everything my doctor told me to do, and I still cannot get pregnant. What went wrong?"

When conception is difficult for you, as it is with these two women, you will need to see a doctor who specializes in fertility problems. Together, you can map out a program that most satisfactorily helps your condition.

PREGNANCY AND MISCARRIAGE: ANTONIA'S STORY

A thirty-one-year-old flight attendant for a large domestic airline, now living in Salt Lake City, Antonia did not know she had endometriosis until one year ago. After reading about the disease in my book *Listen to Your Body,* she wrote asking my advice. Antonia, like many women, probably had endometriosis since her teen years. Now she was going through all the feelings—from disbelief to anger—about endometriosis while facing the difficult task of getting pregnant.

"I want a baby and suddenly it looks like it may not happen and this scares me. I've been married for eight years and I have been pregnant three times. The first time, when I was eighteen, I had an abortion. Six years ago, I had a miscarriage at the end of the first trimester, and the same thing happened a year later. I haven't been able to get pregnant again. Since then, I've been through every fertility test possible.

"I had surgery a year ago for endometriosis. In a two-hour operation, the doctor removed my left ovary and tube because the endometriosis was so bad. He also did a resection of my right ovary and he put dye through my right tube to ensure that it was open. He told me there's no reason why I shouldn't be able to conceive now. He said that pregnancy is the only cure for endometriosis, and he even told me strongly not to come back until I become pregnant! I went to another doctor who advised Danocrine to help get rid of any more endometriosis and improve my chances of having a baby. Is there anything more I can do? What are my chances of having a family?"

Antonia's first doctor may have meant to indicate that she should just relax and take it easy—and that this would help her conceive. Relaxation may be beneficial, but it is not therapeutic at her stage of the disease. Each menstrual cycle increases the chance of further endometrial implantations and complications. Emotional stress focusing on not being able to conceive cannot help either. Antonia's choice to seek a second opinion and to be treated with Danocrine was a wise one.

Dr. Robert Kistner, formerly affiliated with Harvard Medical School and Brigham and Women's Hospital in Boston, and one of the many innovative doctors to make outstanding contributions in the treatment of endometriosis, stated that the chance of getting the disease is greater among women who menstruate cycle after cycle without a break for five years or more.

A higher incidence of miscarriage is a known medical fact among women with endometriosis. Some studies show a high rate of 49 percent of miscarriage for women with mild endometriosis, and about 25 percent in those with moderate to severe cases. One study showed that miscarriage rates declined to 6 percent or less following danazol treatment, depending on the case and whether the medication was given in tandem with surgery or another protocol. Conception, then, may be possible if you have the disease, but carrying a child to full term can be problematic.

This explains, in part, Antonia's crisis. Many women have a hard time believing that endometriosis has such control of their bodies, especially when it impairs a basic function like childbearing. Because endometriosis is a progressive disease, it demands attention at the earliest possible stages to prevent actual damage to internal organs. Antonia will need to be scrupulous in following a healing program set up by her doctor. If she does not conceive after taking Danocrine, I would suggest laser laparoscopy, since this procedure can be used to remove adhesions that women with endometriosis tend to develop. After surgery, if necessary, I would suggest another six months on Danocrine taken along with the endometriosis diet and a vitamin program.

If all else fails, Antonia might once again have a fertility workup. This includes a series of tests such as a pelvic examination, a laparoscopy to determine any tubal, ovarian, or uterine problems resulting from endometriosis, an X ray and ultrasound examination of the uterus, and other routine blood and urine tests to check for hormone levels, anemia, and other factors. It would also be a wise move for Antonia's husband to have a semen analysis, a culture to check for harmful bacteria, and other standard sperm tests. If Antonia proves to be ovulating, if her remaining fallopian tube is free of endometriotic cysts or adhesions and appears to be functioning, and if there are no uterine problems, she might benefit from fertility drugs.

Since women with endometriosis have a more difficult time conceiving, she could be a good candidate for artificial insemination, with her husband's sperm.

How Can Endometriosis Cause Infertility?

What exactly happens to cause infertility in Antonia and other women due to endometriosis?

Even microscopic endometriosis tissue will produce prostaglandins, the hormone that interferes with the release of eggs. It is also thought that endometriosis affects the mechanism that regulates the coordination between the fimbriae—or fingerlike ends of the fallopian tubes, which are intended to "grab" the egg upon its release from the ovary— and the ovary. It is also possible that endometriosis interferes with ovulation itself, often by preventing the eggs from being released from the ovary. Endometriosis can pull internal organs out of line. When this happens around the ovaries, the fimbriated ends of the tubes might not be able to *reach* the eggs as they are expelled from the ovary.

A laparoscopy might reveal that the fallopian tubes are normal in every aspect, but that the uterus is retroverted, or tilted backwards. Often, pregnancy does not occur among endometriosis sufferers who have this condition. One result of uterine retroversion is that the ovaries and tubes can be drawn backward to rest in the cul-de-sac, an area behind the uterus where fluids and organic secretions accumulate. There are always fluids in the abdominal cavity so the organs can move smoothly against each other. When you are standing up, these fluids will lie on the floor of the peritoneal cavity and in the cul-de-sac. However, the woman with endometriosis also produces prostaglandins, secreted by the endometriosis, as well as other secretions doctors have not yet isolated. It is believed that fertility is impeded because these hostile fluids can damage or kill the eggs before they can enter the fallopian tubes.

Ovaries also produce progesterone, the second female hormone. The literal meaning of the word is "for" *(pro)* "gestation," or pregnancy *(gesterone)*. Its production and assimilation in the body relaxes the uterus. This relaxation creates a friendlier environment for the egg to implant itself. It will also lower the level of prostaglandins so there is less cramping, reducing the chance of miscarriage. If the prostaglandin level is high, women might experience more cramping, creating a hostile environment in which the embryo cannot implant itself. Progesterone also prepares the uterus so it can provide a spongy nest for egg implantation and growth. In part, this progesterone emanates from the corpus luteum, the ruptured follicle from which the egg is discharged. If the corpus luteum is not well formed, progesterone is lower, more prostaglandins surge, and contractions might prevent conception or lead to miscarriage.

Some women with premenstrual syndrome who have bad cramping and/or endometriosis along with this cyclical problem are found to have an inadequate luteal phase, which results in a lower progesterone level. The luteal phase is the time span of approximately two weeks from ovulation to menstruation. When this happens, progesterone and estrogen levels decrease rapidly, releasing prostaglandins, which in turn start menstruation. To aid these women in conception, many fertility specialists are recommending natural progesterone suppositories, which are inserted vaginally during the last two weeks of the menstrual cycle. These suppositories melt in the vagina and are absorbed into the bloodstream through the vaginal mucosa. Since natural progesterone doesn't yet come in pill form (it would be destroyed by stomach acids and the liver), the suppository is the most practical method of use.

Another problem, related to egg release and occurring among women with endometriosis, has the estimable name of luteinized unruptured follicle syndrome, or LUF, a condition in which a woman may menstruate regularly and there is "presumed" evidence of ovulation, but it happens *without* the release of the egg from the ovary. Because of various factors, among them the higher prostaglandin levels of endometriosis, the follicle becomes luteinized (that is, it

OVULATION AND FERTILIZATION

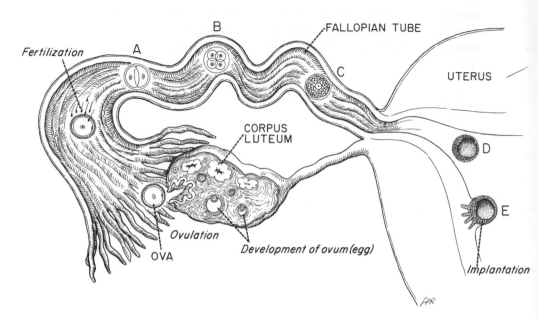

begins to produce progesterone) without apparent ovulation, and the egg becomes trapped and destroyed inside the ovary. In this case, endometriosis needs to be treated with drugs such as Danocrine, and ovulation–inducing fertility drugs will help to create a healthier folli-cle. (The illustration shows ovulation with the release of an egg from the ovary. The egg then moves to the fallopian tube, where fertiliza-tion occurs. If you have endometriosis, the disease may cause the fimbriae, the fingerlike ends of the tubes, to adhere together, or implants can twist and distort the hair-fine tubes out of shape. Such distortions can prevent conception.)

WHAT IS UNEXPLAINED INFERTILITY?

Although the endometriosis in its many forms may affect fertility, there are also other factors, as yet undescribed and so far unknown, which affect whether or not a woman can conceive. It is generally called unexplained infertility.

Studies reveal that no cause can be found for about 10 to 20 percent of all women who cannot have a child. Doctors speculate that the cause or causes, still unidentified, are mysterious only because they escape detection or diagnosis using the methods that are available now. When fertility specialists examine the reasons for a woman not conceiving, they will take many factors into consideration. If a woman has a condition like endometriosis and it has been therapeutically treated in some way—through surgery, hormone treatment, diet, or a combination of these—and there is no conception after about six months, she will need to have a fertility workup to check each fertility factor one by one.

What is this workup? It will include:
• the taking of basal body temperature on a daily basis to help determine if there is ovulation
• a pelvic examination to indicate if there are any organic abnormalities
• a Pap smear to rule out cancer
• if it is indicated, a laparoscopy to determine if there are any pelvic problems
• a hysterosalpingogram, or X ray of the uterus and tubes

Other tests focus on conception itself. A postcoital test requires that a woman be examined immediately following intercourse to check the chemical composition of her cervical mucus and the motility of the sperm in the mucus. Semen analysis is mandatory to rule out problems involving sperm count, sperm shape (morphology), and motility.

Unexplained infertility in women is often caused by endometriosis, which can be confirmed only through laparoscopy. In one study done at the Naval Regional Medical Center in Oakland, California, a team of doctors studied 229 couples who were evaluated for unexplained infertility. Focusing on 24 couples with abnormal findings, unsuspected endometriosis was eventually found in 46 percent of cases. This number is consistent with other reports describing the connection between this disease and fertility—and points up, once again, how insidious this disease can be.

"How do I know if I have some other undiagnosed problem beyond my endometriosis?" In cases of unexplained infertility with completely normal pelvic findings, I suggest that a woman be placed on birth control pills for a few months, to allow a rest from the menstrual cycle. These should be taken in tandem with extra vitamin B complex and B_6. After stopping the birth control pills, she may want to pinpoint the day of ovulation by using a commercially available ovulation predictor kit. The kit allows a woman to test her urine each morning, and a specific indicator in the kit will turn blue twenty-four hours before ovulation occurs. If she takes this advice and still does not conceive within a few months, I believe the next step is 400 or 600 mg of Danocrine on a daily basis for three to four months in case she is in the early stages of microscopic endometriosis. If there is still no conception after this treatment, then she might be a candidate for fertility drugs, *in vitro* fertilization, or the GIFT procedure. I will discuss these techniques very shortly.

Science is always reaching forward, and it is my belief that eventually we will have an answer for unexplained infertility.

QUESTIONS TO ASK YOUR DOCTOR
ABOUT A FERTILITY WORKUP

1. What kind of tests will you be giving me?
2. Is there anything I should or shouldn't do or eat before the tests?
3. What do you think the tests will tell you about my case?
4. Where will you give me these tests? In your office? At a clinic or hospital?
5. Will any of these tests demand an overnight stay?
6. When will you get the results and let me know of them?
7. Will I need to have my husband/boyfriend with me for any test?
8. If so, what should he know and will he need to take time off from work?
9. Will I need to have the tests done a second or third time to confirm any results?
10. How much will these tests cost? Will my health insurance pay for them?

FERTILITY DRUGS: WHAT THEY CAN DO FOR YOU

I received an interesting note from a woman who has just relocated to Columbus, Ohio, where her husband was transferred. Donna, who is twenty-eight years old and has a seven-year-old son, has decided to have another child. She thought the move to another city was a good time to have a baby; she could use her time at home with the baby to settle in for a while before thinking about a part-time career. Donna wrote that she was diagnosed as having severe endometriosis on her right ovary, a moderate amount on her bladder, and some scar tissue around her fallopian tubes from earlier surgery.

Donna has been unable to conceive for a year. She wrote, "First I was put on the birth control pill Norlestrin for three months to suppress the endometriosis. Then I was given 50 mg of Clomid, to be taken from the fifth to the ninth day, and with it, .3 mg of Premarin to induce ovulation. Nothing happened after five months. My doctor said that if I want another baby, the only thing left for me is surgery, to cut away the endometrial masses. This doctor does not believe in Danocrine. What would you suggest?"

Donna's quandary is understandable. She has been put on a program of drugs that did not work for her, and she is at the same place as before spending all that money on medication. Norlestrin is not a treatment of choice for endometriosis now, nor was it ever approved by the FDA for this condition. Norlestrin's formula is based on estrogen and progesterone, which we now know can stimulate the growth of the disease, rather than shrink it. If Donna does not want surgery, she may seek a second opinion from a doctor about the feasibility of taking Danocrine.

Fertility drugs, like Clomid (clomiphene citrate) and the well-known Pergonal (human menopausal gonadotropins), can be given to women with endometriosis, but they need to be dosed on an individual basis. I generally have found, as have other specialists throughout the country, that patients with endometriosis who are given only Clomid have more frequent recurrences of endometriosis. There is no conclusive answer as to why this might be. Clomid tends to work best for women who have polycystic ovarian syndrome, a condition that may interrupt the normal process of ovulation each month.

Clomid, like Danocrine, is an "antihormone," although its functions differ greatly. Clomid lowers the estrogen level during the five days it is taken before midmonth ovulation occurs. When the drug is stopped, there is a spurt of estrogen back into the body. The estrogen will begin the triggering cycle to the hypothalamus. That gland will, in turn, release the luteinizing hormone, causing ovulation. Pergonal, often used in combination with Clomid, has a separate function: stimulating the ovaries to develop the egg-containing follicles, so that when ovulation occurs, *several* eggs might be released. Pergonal's origin has a slight ring of medieval alchemy to it, having been first made in Italy from the purified urine of menopausal nuns. Postmenopausal women tend to produce large amounts of LH and FSH, which is excreted in their urine. Pergonal, supplied from such sources, has been instrumental in helping many childless women conceive.

Because Pergonal is a more powerful drug than Clomid, giving it to a very young woman who is more likely to be more fertile will produce a greater number of eggs and increase the chance of multiple births. In the case of a woman with endometriosis, the production of several eggs might not result in multiple births, since some eggs have a higher chance of being damaged or destroyed.

Pergonal, unlike Clomid, was originally used for women who did not menstruate, who had lengthy menstrual periods, or who never ovulated, but who had a great store of eggs which needed a stimulating hormone to help release them. A similar situation tends to exist among women with endometriosis who have difficulty in conceiving: they, too, might benefit from a stimulating hormone to help trigger egg release. The best time for a program of fertility drugs for these women is right after Danocrine treatment, when prostaglandin levels are lowest.

Pergonal is best administered in combination with Clomid and HCG (human chorionic gonadotropin, a drug similar to the brain hormone LH, which brings on ovulation) in a sequence of varying doses for almost twelve days. Then it is time for you to see your doctor again. He can give you a sonogram (ultrasound) to see how many eggs you have produced. On day thirteen, HCG (LH) is administered by injection to trigger ovulation. If ultrasound reveals that there are more than five or six *mature* follicles, your doctor may not give HCG. Otherwise, HCG is given and ovulation occurs the next day. This method will only occasionally result in multiple births. Because of *in vitro* techniques—fertilizing eggs outside the uterus and implanting them back in the uterus or tube—doctors have learned more about the capabilities of these drugs in producing and releasing eggs and effectively helping women with conception.

Another fertility drug, analogous to Pergonal, is being used for women with endometriosis who may also suffer from polycystic ovaries: Metrodin (urofollitropin). Although it, too, is extracted from the urine of postmenopausal women, unlike Pergonal, Metrodin is pure FSH (follicle-stimulating hormone), whereas Pergonal combines FSH with LH (luteinizing hormone). Metrodin is given by injection on a daily basis for about eleven days. This is followed by HCG on day twelve, which should render a woman fertile within 24 to 36 hours. It is best to avoid having intercourse until at least one day from the time of injection of HCG to ensure, for one thing, a man's higher sperm count on day thirteen.

My advice to Donna would be to undergo laser surgery after taking Danocrine to clear away some of her adhesions and obstructive endometrial masses, followed by a program of Clomid and Pergonal. Laser surgery followed by Danocrine for a few months might help, to remove microscopic implants. Yet there is no guarantee that endometriosis will not return. No doctor can promise that. However, Donna is still young enough to take these various programs, one step at a time. Eventually, she may have the second child she wants. My only warning to her is this: should she decide she wants a larger family, and she conceives her second child, I would recommend that she try to conceive a third time as soon after the birth of the baby as possible. With endometriosis, there is always a chance that it will return. Couple that with the aging factor, and Donna's chances of conceiving would be even lower than before.

Is *in Vitro* Fertilization or GIFT the Answer for You?

In vitro fertilization, much in the news, has improved enormously in recent years. A few years ago, it was the most difficult and complicated, if not the most expensive, tool to help produce conception. Although *in vitro* techniques have been improved, resorting to them should be the final recourse, since it is costly and not every case is successful.

Who is a good candidate for *in vitro* or the GIFT procedure? If you have endometriosis or unexplained infertility, you must be fully evaluated in the fashion described earlier in this chapter, including basal temperature and X rays of the uterus and tubes, to be sure that you have a menstrual cycle and are ovulating. If you seem to be ovulating (or do so after taking fertility drugs) but still do not conceive, and in spite of artificial insemination you do not get pregnant, the next step for you may be *in vitro* fertilization or GIFT, an acronym for gamete intra-fallopian tube transfer, a variation of *in vitro* fertilization.

GIFT is similar to *in vitro* fertilization in that it shares some of the same technology in retrieving eggs. However, as developed by Dr. Ricardo H. Asch, who in 1984 was experimenting with such a technique at the University of Texas, fertilization takes place inside the body rather than outside it. With *in vitro* fertilization, an egg is removed from the ovary, fertilized by sperm, and incubated *outside* the body (specifically, in a glass petri dish). Then two days later, the embryo is placed in the uterus. The GIFT procedure was a solution to the problem of egg failing to meet sperm at a normal site of fertilization—the fallopian tube. Under normal conditions, the egg will be released from the ovary, and if it is fertilized by sperm, it will divide several times as it travels down the tube. After a few days, the fertilized egg, now an embryo, enters the uterus and implants itself on the wall of the womb. The GIFT technique artificially duplicates this process, placing egg and sperm in the fallopian tube, where conception can occur naturally. The eggs are first aspirated during a laparoscopy and examined under a microscope. If they are healthy, they are then mixed with sperm before being placed in the tube.

Dr. Asch speculated that pregnancy would be more successful if the body prepared itself for pregnancy as it happened—that is, from fertilization of the egg in the tube to its implantation in the womb. *In vitro* fertilization has now taken a back seat to the GIFT technique, since the former has proved to be not as successful a mode of fertilization.

These techniques may offer hope for some women with fertility problems related to endometriosis. Recall that one result of the disease is that it can prevent release of the egg from the ovary. Doctors have also seen that prostaglandin levels might interfere with sperm motility. The GIFT technique especially bypasses these preventatives to conception, since there are no prostaglandins inside the fallopian tubes to interfere with conception. For the GIFT procedure to be feasible, at least *one* fallopian tube must be normal and there must be evidence of ovulation. Of course, a specialist in the technique will need to determine if the procedure could work for you. If both tubes are damaged and at least one cannot be surgically corrected, then *in vitro* fertilization would be the last course of action.

Should you choose such innovative techniques, you would be asked to follow a simple step-by-step process. Following a physical examination of both you and your partner, you would be given fertility drugs, such as Clomid and Pergonal, to stimulate the development of ovarian follicles and increase the chances of producing and retrieving *ripened* eggs from the ovary. This is followed by a sonogram to see if the follicles are developing satisfactorily. Then you would be admitted into a clinic or hospital for a laparoscopy, during which time the eggs would be retrieved, or aspirated, from the ovary.

A newer technique for egg retrieval through the use of ultrasound technique eliminates the need for laparoscopy or a brief hospital stay. Developed in Denmark, ultrasonic egg retrieval is being used increasingly in some centers for *in vitro* fertilization *only,* and not for the GIFT procedure. Basically an office procedure, ultrasound is employed as a guide to pinpoint the location of ovarian follicles. The doctor then inserts a long needle through the abdominal wall or the vagina, punctures the follicles, and aspirates the eggs. To keep the process a painless one, the patient is given an intravenous painkiller and local anesthetic. Although it is, in a way, a simpler system of egg retrieval, not every woman having *in vitro* fertilization is a candidate for this technique.

Once retrieved, the eggs are examined under a microscope. If they look healthy, they will be mixed with sperm—usually taken from your partner about two or three hours earlier, examined for quality, and specially washed before being mixed with the eggs.

If you are undergoing the GIFT procedure, you will be placed under anesthesia for the entire procedure—both for egg retrieval and for the final phase: the placement of eggs and sperm in the fallopian tube, where, it is hoped, fertilization will take place. After about ten days, a pregnancy test is conducted to see if conception has, indeed, occurred.

So far, there has been no increase in the incidence of fetal abnormalities following these techniques, although there is a greater percentage of multiple births. Estimates are that about 20 percent are twin births, and a much smaller percentage of women have triplets. In my experience, it is rare for a woman with endometriosis to have twins or triplets. The nature of the disease and its effect on the body may be less likely to support the birth of more than one child at a time. Of course, it also depends on how many eggs a doctor chooses to implant at one time. The point in mixing sperm with more than one egg is to optimize the odds of fertilization using this costly and lengthy procedure.

Using these techniques, clinics have reported a range of successes as high as 40 percent. This success rate is based on pregnancy rates after a *series* of such fertilizations, not on a one-time try, since women infrequently conceive on the first attempt. Most fertility specialists will advise couples to wait a few months before trying again if no conception takes place.

In vitro and GIFT are extraordinary in their ability to facilitate conception. They can set up the situation that makes pregnancy possible, but there is still a wide margin of error. While *in vitro* and GIFT can offer the miracle of birth to women with endometriosis, these procedures are at this point expensive. Beyond the issue of cost, some women can feel great emotional stress during the procedure, and worry about the results.

Because the probability of conception with endometriosis is reduced, you will want to be treated by the best practitioners in the field. Be sure that the doctor you choose is a highly respected fertility expert. Fertility clinics have cropped up around the country and have become big business. Investigate your doctor's credentials before signing any consent forms for the procedure.

It is my belief that these techniques will be used more and more in the future. Right now, they *could* be the answer for women with endometriosis.

CAN ENDOMETRIOSIS INCREASE THE CHANCES OF ECTOPIC PREGNANCIES?

Ectopic pregnancy is the result of normal fertilization occurring in an abnormal site, a phenomenon limited to humans. Ectopic pregnancy describes a condition in which a fertilized egg does not travel from the tube to the uterus, as it should, but, instead, implants itself in the fallopian tube, on an ovary, or somewhere else in the abdominal cavity. About 1 percent of all pregnancies are ectopic, and statistics show they are on the rise.

I received a letter from a woman in Iowa who has a number of problems related to endometriosis. Nina, who is twenty-seven years old and has been married for seven years, has been in and out of hospitals over the last two years in an effort to clear up endometriosis and eventually have a family. She wrote to me about this problem:

"After finally getting pregnant ten months ago, it turned out to be an ectopic pregnancy. My husband and I really want a baby, but now I'm getting worried. I have been having pain off and on for five months on the right side, the site of the ectopic pregnancy. This pain radiates to my lower back. A recent hysterosalpingogram revealed that my tubes are hanging toward the back and the right tube is wrapped around toward the left side. I went in for microsurgery and the doctor told me she removed as many adhesions as she could.

"I need to mention that after two years of pain, doctors keep telling me that I am just a 'nervous type.' I finally realized what's been wrong with me when I read your book and then asked my doctor for a laparoscopy. I had endometriosis. When I conceived, I knew from the symptoms that it was an ectopic pregnancy, but my doctor at first told me to stop worrying. As I feared, I had a tubal pregnancy. I've always been right when it comes to my body, and my intuition tells me that I may not be able to have a child normally. What are my chances for conceiving again and avoiding a tubal pregnancy? Can you please advise me on this?"

At one time, it was felt that infection, such as pelvic inflammatory disease, damaged the tubes, making it difficult for normal pregnancy to occur. However, doctors are now concluding that a disease like endometriosis may in some part be responsible. During retrograde menstruation, implants may get stuck in the tubes and form obstructions.

Women with endometriosis are advised to see their doctors as soon as pregnancy is discovered. An early sonogram, taken at the fifth week of pregnancy, can ensure that the amniotic sac is developing in the uterus. If it is a tubal pregnancy, exploratory surgery and removal of the conceptus must be done immediately to prevent bursting of the fallopian tube. After that, I would recommend Danocrine and a good diet for four to six months before trying conception again.

Nina shares a problem common to women who are higher-risk candidates for infertility related to endometriosis. She needs to be carefully monitored, after a program of danazol therapy. Because the incidence of ectopic pregnancy is as high as 25 percent in women with endometriosis, women who have had a tubal pregnancy should undergo a hysterosalpingogram (X ray of the uterus and tubes) before conceiving again. The X ray will determine if there is any tubal damage that would precipitate a chance for a second tubal pregnancy. If this happens, the only chance for having a child depends on *in vitro* fertilization.

DOES ENDOMETRIOSIS AFFECT THE CHANCE OF CONCEIVING A BOY OR GIRL?

A patient with endometriosis called to say she'd heard that the disease can affect whether or not she will give birth to a boy. Marcia has been trying to conceive for three months after having laser surgery and six months of danazol therapy. Although she would be happy just to have a child, she wondered if it was true: "Could endometriosis determine the sex of the baby? Why would it happen?"

Marcia sounded disbelieving, but a recent study on patients who have had successful pregnancies with mild endometriosis did show an interesting discrepancy between the rates of live male and female births. The study, undertaken by Dr. Mark F. Severino of the State University of New York at the Buffalo School of Medicine, disclosed that there was a higher rate of females born to such women after treatment for endometriosis—approximately two times more girls were born than boys. Other studies, however, do not show a greater proportion of the birth of girls over boys.

Marcia's question "Why would it happen?" cannot yet be fully and precisely answered. We do know that sperm carrying the X chromosomes (for a female) are larger and hardier than the sperm carrying the male marker (or Y) and that while the "males" are smaller, they are faster swimmers. It may be that sperm containing the X chromosome can better survive a hostile environment. Prostaglandins produced by endometriotic tissue in large amounts can act as a spermicide. In his study, Dr. Severino postulated that there is "selective ingestion of sperm carrying the Y chromosome by pelvic macrophages, which might explain this imbalance in the secondary sex ratio." Again, there is no clue as to why these immune system fighters would react to the chemistry of Y sperm and destroy some of them.

Fertility specialists have found that if a woman conceives right at the time of ovulation, her chances are greater for having a boy. The Y-chromosome sperm, being smaller and faster swimmers, can also move more quickly through the egg membrane to fertilize it. However, if a woman has sexual intercourse a few days before ovulation, these tend to die off and her chances of bearing a daughter increase, if only because X-chromosome sperm tend to live longer. *In vitro* fertilization and the GIFT procedure tend to favor boys, since fresh and healthy sperm is mixed with the egg at ovulation.

If you want a baby and you have endometriosis, there are options open for you. The first step is to select a doctor who specializes in endometriosis and fertility problems. This is in your own best interest. Specialists know what is happening in their field, and this one is rapidly changing. They speak with colleagues all over the world, exchange information, visit clinics, do comparative studies, and concentrate on this subject alone. A specialist can evaluate your case on an individual basis and devise a plan of action—from preparing your body so it is more capable of bearing a child to determining how you may best conceive, be it naturally, through artificial insemination, or by *in vitro* fertilization. A specialist can also tell the endometriosis patient what her best chances are for conception with the GIFT method.

CHAPTER 13

Hysterectomy:
It's Not a Cure for Endometriosis

ONCE considered the only cure for endometriosis, hysterectomy is now being looked at from a different perspective. Many women wonder if such radical surgery isn't the shortsighted view of how to treat the disease.

Those who are entirely opposed to this operation believe that it should be done only when it is clearly lifesaving surgery, and at no other time. Since complications from endometriosis are rarely life-threatening, opponents of hysterectomy paint a damning picture of how few doctors respect women's bodies, citing the frequency of hysterectomies. This is strong stuff, and in a way, it is a correct assessment.

Here is a good example of how women can be pressured into having a hysterectomy. A woman with endometriosis came to see me for a second opinion. Her doctor had suggested a hysterectomy, not only because she had endometriosis but for two other reasons as well. "I've been dealing with endometriosis for about fifteen years now," Georgette told me. "I've also got a uterine fibroid that is about the size of an apricot and gives me problems about once a year. My doctor told me that I needed a hysterectomy for three reasons: First, he argued, I was forty-five and too old to have any more children, so why did I need a uterus? Second, I had endometriosis, and third, I had a fibroid that caused bleeding and pain once in a while. The doctor's rationale for surgery was that a hysterectomy would prevent a recurrence of the fibroids and probably would help the endometriosis.

"Quite honestly," Georgette said, "I felt insulted. Although I have had some trouble with endometriosis even after two years on Danocrine, the disease has not severely damaged my uterus or ovaries. It's true I don't want any more children, but that is no justification for major surgery such as this. And removing my uterus to prevent fibroids from possibly growing larger or perhaps growing new ones is, to me, tantamount to decapitating me to prevent the possibility of my being bothered by headaches in the future!"

Georgette's story is not unusual, but the good news is that doctors are easing up on their tendency to perform this operation when it is not absolutely a life-or-death issue. Nonetheless, this is an emotionally loaded decision for nearly every woman. Very few happily undergo this operation and give up their organs with a sense of relief.

BE A PARTNER IN THE DECISION-MAKING

The woman with endometriosis, I have found, always thinks about her chances of being a candidate for hysterectomy. It is a word that tends to come up a lot during medical examinations and in conversations with other women. A woman worries if the disease will progress to a point where her doctor will recommend this surgery. If she agrees to the operation, she wonders if she will later find that it was not necessary. On the one hand, her doctor, the expert, is telling her that it will stop her pain. On the other, women's groups and other health-related organizations inform her that hysterectomy is not the answer. It is here that she may feel ambushed by fear, guilt, and confusion. What should she do?

Making a decision about hysterectomy requires information and a cool head. The crucial thing to know is that every woman has control of her destiny—she need not sign away her organs carte blanche when she checks into the hospital. This kind of passivity was more common twenty years ago. I reiterate it because I find that women still defer to others when it comes to making choices about their own health.

We barely need to be reminded of how women have changed over the last two decades, not only in terms of what they can expect in life but in how they have connected with their bodies. The woman of the

1980s investigates her options carefully with regard to her life and health. Yet, paradoxically, many women will agree to hysterectomy *because it is presented as a life-or-death decision.*

Statistics tell us that nearly 80 percent of all surgery is optional, or elective, while the remaining 20 percent requires the lifesaving decision to operate. In most cases, a hysterectomy *does not* fall within this latter range, although there is no question that a woman with, for example, uterine cancer or untreatable uterine damage would be advised to have this operation to save her life and protect her health. What is most relevant is that hysterectomy is the *most performed* major surgery in America. Are all these hysterectomies necessary?

Though hysterectomy may have been performed too freely two decades ago, doctors had fewer feasible alternatives than they do now for stopping the terrible pain and damage of endometriosis. As you know, Danocrine, the "antihormone" responsible for melting away endometriotic masses, was not available until thirteen years ago, and the gonadotropin-releasing hormone analogs, or agonists, are only very recent contributions to drug therapy for the disease. Video-laseroscopy is still newer as a form of treatment.

THE UTERUS: MORE IMPORTANT TO WELL-BEING THAN IT SEEMS

Most damaging, years ago, were commonly held opinions about hysterectomy, the purpose of the uterus, and the long-term side effects of such surgery. Two decades ago, doctors were more likely to operate under the misguided opinion that the uterus had no value other than its mechanical function of bearing a child. A woman with severe endometriosis or uterine fibroids would have been given a hysterectomy with very little thought to the tremendous physiological and psychological aftershock.

Twenty years ago, too, women tended to take the word of doctors as gospel. They believed what they were told when doctors promised them that hysterectomy would not change their lives. In fact, some were told not only that they would be relieved of pain along with their reproductive organs but that they would be freer to enjoy sex. In some cases this was true. For many others, however, sexual pleasure was diminished and other unpleasant symptoms became an overwhelming reality. These symptoms were hot flashes, depression, weight gain, and the risk of osteoporosis, among others.

Despite all the alternative treatments that are available now, many doctors still hold to the old-fashioned view that hysterectomy is the final answer for endometriosis. Such doctors are of the opinion that by removing the uterus alone or by removing the ovaries and tubes as well, they are excising the source of the disease and eliminating the chance of its recurrence. We know differently. Endometriosis may exist *microscopically,* not just in host reproductive organs, but in the bladder, bowel, and even in the lungs. Moreover, if the woman who has had her uterus *and* her ovaries removed is given estrogen replacement therapy (ERT) immediately after surgery, the disease may regrow and become as disruptive as before. I have treated many women who are, in fact, doubly suffering: they are trying to cope with the recurrent pain of endometriosis along with the shocking symptoms of sudden menopause caused by hysterectomy.

As it stands now, hysterectomy is the most performed major operation for American women between the ages of fifteen and forty-four years of age, with the average age for this elective surgery being thirty-five years. According to published figures as reported by HERS (Hysterectomy Educational Resources and Services), an organization that gathers information on hysterectomy, its risks, complications, and alternatives, 35 million women have had hysterectomies. In 1985 alone, figures for this radical surgery reached about 1 million; of them, over half the women also had their ovaries removed, even if these organs were not diseased.

Many doctors, like me, do not believe in performing a hysterectomy unless it is lifesaving surgery and/or the last course of action. Although numbers vary widely, it is reasonable to say that *at least 25 to 30 percent of hysterectomies are unnecessary,* and I know gynecologists who estimate that this number may be as high as 70 to 90 percent! Nevertheless, a documented statistic tells us that one-half of all American women who live to sixty-five years old will reach this age having had a hysterectomy.

Hysterectomy as a panacea for endometriosis or other problems of the reproductive tract has come under closer scrutiny these last few years. It is not a simple operation and the feelings connected to it are often complex. Women should become more informed on this issue and feel free to refuse this surgery, until they get a second or third opinion. It is interesting to note that since the number of unnecessary hysterectomies has reached immense proportions, most insurance carriers now require a second opinion.

HYSTERECTOMY: WHAT IS IT?

Hysterectomy may be divided into five separate procedures.

Technically, a partial, or subtotal, hysterectomy involves the surgical removal of the uterus only; no other organ is excised. When a surgeon performs a total, or complete, hysterectomy, he is removing the uterus and cervix. (See illustration below.) The cervix, or "mouth of the womb," is the lower portion of the uterus, which protrudes into the vagina. About an inch in diameter, the cervix can vary in firmness as well as change its position slightly during sexual arousal or at stages of the menstrual cycle. The cervix may be excised for a number of reasons, such as severe infection and precancerous or cancerous conditions.

The third approach is more radical and involves the removal of the uterus and both ovaries. This is called a total hysterectomy with a bilateral oophorectomy. A total hysterectomy with a bilateral salpingo-oophorectomy means the uterus, cervix, ovaries, and tubes are removed. Finally, there is a radical hysterectomy, used extensively in

Total Hysterectomy

Before

After

199

cases of uterine or cervical cancer. Here the uterus, cervix, part of the vagina, and some of the tissue surrounding the uterus is removed. The ovaries and tubes are also usually, not always, removed in this procedure.

Because each type of hysterectomy is different, any woman discussing this operation with her doctor urgently needs to clarify the terms—and what will be happening to her. If the doctor is talking in shorthand, saying it's just a simple hysterectomy and telling you not to worry, do not accept such offhand explanations. You must know *precisely* what will be taken out and what will be left in. There is a great difference in how you will feel (and recover) after a uterus is removed compared with how you will feel when you are thrown into sudden surgical menopause with removal of the ovaries and tubes.

A total hysterectomy with excision of the ovaries is not a sensible choice for a woman in her reproductive years. Without ovaries, there is a drastic drop of estrogen and progesterone levels, signaling abrupt "change of life" symptoms, such as hot flashes, metabolic changes like weight gain, loss of sex drive, and the threat of irreversible osteoporosis. In the last few years, new attention has been focused on the increased prevalence of heart disease among women who have had hysterectomies, with or without the removal of ovaries. Studies have been undertaken to investigate the hormone prostacyclin, which is produced by uterine tissue even after menopause. There is a possible link between prostacyclin, a known vasodilator, or substance that dilates veins and helps strengthen the arteries, and the prevention of cardiovascular disease.

If you are a woman who has not yet reached natural menopause, and you have been told you need a hysterectomy, find a doctor who will do his best to preserve the ovaries, if they are healthy. Unless there is bowel or uterine cancer, for example, with a high risk of the disease spreading to the ovaries, which can be fatal, perhaps at least one ovary can be retained. There are circumstances, too, where ovarian endometriotic cysts have damaged portions of these organs. A good surgeon will try to save what he can of the healthy ovarian tissue, so it can still function.

When is a hysterectomy called for and how do you know what should be removed? Hysterectomy is a last resort to consider—only when all other treatments fail and you are still suffering. I think these two stories, told from two different points of view, might help you understand the problem.

HYSTERECTOMY FOR ENDOMETRIOSIS: PRO AND CON

Con: "Hysterectomy Nearly Ruined My Life"

Not every woman elects to have a hysterectomy and some are not even forewarned by their surgeons that they will be undergoing this procedure. Hysterectomy due to complications of endometriosis can come as a surprise to the woman who thought she was going in for a simple removal of a cyst. There are cases, too, where other unexpected complications from hysterectomy are shocking. A thirty-three-year-old woman from Georgia wrote me of her sad plight. Penny, who has been married for thirteen years and has twin girls, described her experience:

"I had signs of endometriosis for some time without a diagnosis. By the time a definitive diagnosis was made, the disease was in an extreme state. It covered my tubes and ovaries on both sides and the floor of my pelvis. It also had grown over my bowel. After taking Danocrine for three and a half months and still being in severe pain, it was decided that I should have a complete 'clean-out.' I got a second opinion and this doctor said the same thing: I should have a hysterectomy to remove my ovaries and tubes.

"I had the surgery, and I came out of anesthesia with a colostomy!" Penny continued. "Fortunately, the colostomy was reversed six months later. After surgery, I was placed on hormone replacement therapy. It's been nearly three years and I've just been taken off hormone replacement. The doctor found that endometriosis has returned and he put me on Depo-Provera.

"I think I made a mistake in having a hysterectomy. I feel ill taking these hormones. I am tired all the time. Sometimes I get anxiety attacks and start crying. I've gained weight that I can't take off. I'm grateful for a loving husband and thankful that I had my daughters before the disease struck so badly. But I am really angry about what I feel was the needless removal of my organs. What can I do?"

Penny's frustration and pain from endometriosis is understandable, as is the shock of waking up from surgery with a colostomy. (In brief, this operation is often performed on patients with cancer of the bowel or a perforated bowel. Surgeons reroute the bowel so it drains outside the body, into a colostomy bag.) I feel that if Penny had been given Danocrine for a longer period of time to disintegrate her adhesions and endometrial growths, she would have noticed a vast improvement and avoided this drastic operation. Although Danocrine is most often given for about six months, as noted in chapter 10, severe cases of endometriosis may demand a more aggressive approach. Since her endometriosis was so extensive, it was obvious that she needed at least a year on the drug. By then it would have melted away some of the larger areas of growth, making laser surgery the next possibility.

It is my opinion that a surgeon unfamiliar with extensive endometriosis operated on her bowel to free endometrial tissue and adhesions that bound the bowel. Such adhesions can complicate surgery. Luckily, the colostomy was able to be reversed. Penny is at a difficult point now: estrogen replacement given too soon after surgery was probably responsible for the regrowth of the endometriosis. Remember, estrogen causes endometriosis to flourish. Therefore, it is deemed advisable to wait at least one year following surgery before starting a woman on hormone replacement. During these twelve months or so, the body's naturally reduced estrogen level gives endometriotic implants a chance to shrink.

Since Penny has had a total hysterectomy with removal of the ovaries and tubes, she could now benefit from a low dosage of Danocrine (200–400 mg daily) for six to nine months. Then Penny will probably need to take a very low dosage estrogen replacement drug, until she reaches the age for natural menopause.

Pro: "Hysterectomy Was a Good Choice for Me"

This story is an ironic one. Thirty-two years old at the time, a mother of three children, and a career woman, Annette believed that a hysterectomy would end the pain of endometriosis and she *insisted on* surgery, although her doctor did not think it was in order at all. As Annette tells it, her story goes this way:

"I was diagnosed as having endometriosis six years ago, right after the birth of my third child," she said. "It finally cleared up the mystery of all the pain I'd been having for years. Then an ovarian cyst ruptured and I had to have emergency surgery. At the same time, I had my uterus suspended and some nerves cut.

"Instead of getting better, things got worse. I had an enlarged uterus and unbelievable pain and heavy bleeding," she continued. "I felt so bad, I couldn't have sex, I was barely a mother to my children, and life was hardly livable. I went to two doctors who both said hysterectomy was the only answer. That bothered me a lot. A hysterectomy at twenty-nine years of age? This sounded drastic to me.

"Then I went to another doctor who I heard was opposed to hysterectomy. He put me on Danocrine and I took it on and off for three years. It helped somewhat, but the drug made me feel depressed and I still had pain in the one remaining ovary. Then I started to hemorrhage. I wanted a hysterectomy, to be free of the cramps, pain, and bleeding. My doctor wouldn't do it, so I went back to the first doctor, and he did it a week later.

"I felt about a hundred times better the day after surgery," Annette said. "And I believe I had no *real* choice about whether or not to have a hysterectomy, even if one doctor was against it. I was in severe pain for years and disabled by bleeding. Keeping my uterus seemed less critical to me than ending these problems—they were just ruining my life. I still have one ovary, so my hormone levels are normal. Most of all, I feel I wasted time when my husband and children saw me debilitated and in pain for years.

"I think this kind of surgery is a personal matter. I am usually happy about my decision to have a hysterectomy, but there are moments when I am ambivalent about it. I have come to understand that this ambivalence is normal. There are times when I feel sad knowing I could never have another child. There are times when I fear that there could be a chance that my remaining ovary will be destroyed by endometriosis and will have to be removed. Then I remember how much pain I was in every day and I *know* I did the right thing for me."

Although she worries about endometriosis spreading to this organ, Annette is generally optimistic. She is attuned to the possible symptoms resulting from hysterectomy that might affect her, such as weight gain and diminished sex drive, but thus far, she has not experienced these reactions. (In fact, since she is finally free of persistent pain, she feels an increased sex drive.) One factor in her favor is a functioning ovary that is supplying enough estrogen and progesterone for her needs. Annette is lucky. Her hysterectomy did not put her into a traumatic state of sudden and premature menopause, and she is feeling healthy.

These cases are dissimilar, but both women were suffering from symptoms of endometriosis that were difficult to live with. Was hysterectomy really the answer for Annette and Penny? The indicators for hysterectomy in cases of endometriosis are:

• when Danocrine or other hormonal therapies do not work and the woman is suffering from debilitating pain

• when a woman does not respond to laser surgery or conservative surgery

• when more than one endometriosis specialist evaluates the case and feels a hysterectomy will help

Even then, it *may or may not* be the answer. As I have stated, hysterectomy should be the last resort, and ideally done at an age when a woman has completed childbearing and is closer to natural menopause.

HYSTERECTOMIES: WHO IS A CANDIDATE?

Other than being the last resort for women with endometriosis, a hysterectomy might be recommended for the following reasons:

• cancer or precancerous lesions of the uterus, ovaries, and fallopian tubes

• untreatable uterine damage that has been precipitated by a severe infection

• surgical trauma that may happen during an abortion or from complications during childbirth in which bleeding cannot be controlled

• exceedingly large fibroids (sometimes the weight of a full-term baby, up to seven or eight pounds) which are too difficult or dangerous to remove through a myomectomy, a surgical removal of tumors from the uterus

Since most hysterectomies are rarely done on an emergency basis, no woman need feel pressured to sign away her organs. There should be a "period of grace" before the decision to go into surgery. This is a good time to seek a second or third opinion about the operation and its effect on a woman's future. Talking it over with counselors and friends offers a chance to hear about the experience of others, garner information, and rally support. You may also write to HERS (Hysterectomy Educational Resources and Services) or the Center for Climacteric Studies at the University of Florida in Gainesville (see appendix for addresses) for further information that can help you make the right decision. Again, there is a small cross section of women who see their future in another light. For them, hysterectomy offers permanent birth control measures and "freedom" from bearing more children than they want. A partial hysterectomy—or removal of the uterus only—is their choice of irreversible contraceptive measures. Most women would not opt for hysterectomy over tubal sterilization as a means of birth control. Most women, in fact, would not understand the reasoning behind such a drastic choice; nevertheless, some women do ask their doctors to perform this unneeded surgery on them. I do not under any circumstances advise hysterectomy in this instance.

HOW IS A HYSTERECTOMY PERFORMED?

"Is hysterectomy always major abdominal surgery?" women ask. The answer is no. Hysterectomies may be done in one of two ways: vaginally or abdominally. Typically, a vaginal hysterectomy is chosen when the uterus is small and not unduly enlarged by fibroids or endometriosis. If there are adhesions attaching the uterus to other pelvic organs, such as the bowel, or if there is scar tissue from previous operations, however, a vaginal hysterectomy is ruled out. It is less common for women with endometriosis to have a vaginal hysterectomy, often because there are too many adhesions and it is more difficult to remove the uterus through this route. Doctors have also found that women who have had no children or who have borne only one child do not have sufficiently stretched vaginas to allow a vaginal hysterectomy.

If it is indicated, a vaginal hysterectomy will take this course: A speculumlike instrument is inserted into the vagina and a light is shone into the operational field. *No abdominal incision* is required. Rather, the doctor holds the cervix in place with a special surgical tool. Then he makes an incision at the top of the vagina into the abdominal cavity. All ligaments and blood vessels are severed and tied, and the uterus (or uterus, ovaries, and tubes, depending on the case) is removed by drawing it out through the vagina. A vaginal hysterectomy means faster recovery with less risk of adhesions. Sometimes abdominal hysterectomy is the wiser and safer procedure, since vaginal hysterectomies require the doctor to work in a very narrow field—through an incision in the vagina. An abdominal hysterectomy is done either through a Pfannenstiel, or bikini-line, incision, a cut made just below the top edge of the pubic hairline, or through a vertical incision made between the navel and the pubic bone, exposing the abdominal cavity. There he can excise the uterus with all its ligaments and, if it is indicated, the ovaries and tubes. Women undergoing an abdominal hysterectomy will need at least six to eight days in the hospital following the operation, though recovery time will vary from patient to patient.

Immediate complications from hysterectomy are few. Death from such surgery is very rare: about one or two patients in every thousand. Infections may set in, especially among women undergoing abdominal hysterectomies, but a skillful surgeon can control these infections with antibiotics. Some blood loss is very common during hysterectomy, especially for the woman with extensive adhesions and severe endometriosis, and blood transfusions are often required. It is important that a woman seek out a skillful surgeon and endometriosis specialist for this type of delicate surgery.

RECOVERING FROM A HYSTERECTOMY

When surgery is performed by a skilled surgeon, you should lose very little blood. The use of hydrocortisone and antibiotics during the surgical procedure reduces the chances of adhesions and eliminates infections. Recovery should then follow this course:

- **Expect some pain and bleeding for several days. This is not uncommon for hysterectomy.**
- **You will not be given solid food for two or three days. Instead, you will be fed intravenously for this amount of time.**
- **A bloated feeling is not unusual. Some women feel an abdominal pressure from an increase in gas.**
- **You should be able to leave the hospital five to eight days after surgery, depending on your individual recovery rate.**
- **Stay at home and get plenty of rest during the next week. Do not do any strenuous physical work, lift any heavy weights, or otherwise place yourself in a physically stressful situation.**
- **When you return home, resume the suggested pre-operative vitamin regimen to strengthen your immune system.**
- **See your doctor two or three weeks after surgery for a follow-up examination. He will advise you as to how you are healing and when he thinks you can resume your normal life-style. In most cases, women can return to work three to seven weeks after surgery.**

AFTEREFFECTS OF HYSTERECTOMY

Rita was twenty-eight years old, working for a large construction company as an office manager. She was about forty pounds over-weight. Rita told me that after two years of "giving up on myself," she was fired with a new determination to change her life following a hysterectomy performed because of complications from endo-metriosis. What happened? Rita told me:

"I had terrible menstrual cramps from the time I was fourteen years old. When I was twenty-three, the doctor told me I had endometriosis and to take the strongest birth control pill on the market. I took one every day with no stopping," she said. "After three months, he told me to take *four pills a day*. My nerves were a wreck and I gained twenty pounds. My body literally revolted against this hormone treatment, and I went through nine tortured weeks of cramps.

"Four months later, at the age of twenty-five, I had a complete hysterectomy. It took me one year to heal completely. I was depressed, had hot flashes, and started to gain more weight. Then I had to adjust to hormone replacement. At that point I was labeled 'cured' by my doctor. Having a hysterectomy at twenty-five was quite traumatic, and no one can understand what I have gone through except other women like me. Now, finally, I'm ready to lose weight and start over. I don't believe I should have had this operation. It's too late now for me, but please make this problem more public."

Rita's case is a sad tale that ends hopefully. It was unfortunate that her doctor overdosed her on oral contraceptives that she did not tolerate well. The high estrogen content of "the strongest birth control pill" was probably instrumental in encouraging the growth of endo-metriosis. Danocrine and conservative surgery might have been a far wiser option than a hysterectomy on a young woman whose ovaries were basically unaffected by the disease.

Her reaction to the operation, though, and the accompanying sense of depression are typical of such women. Many doctors overlook the psychological aspects of such surgery. It is my feeling that women would help themselves if they first spoke to counselors or specialized women's groups comprised of former hysterectomy patients or health care professionals, such as an organization like HERS, who can advise a woman on managing her symptoms and dealing with the finality of surgery.

In one study concentrating on the aftereffects of such surgery, it was

207

found that abdominal hysterectomies may produce hernias, a result of poorly healed wounds. Some women who had vaginal hysterectomies were discovered to suffer from a vaginal enterocele, or a portion of the bowel protruding into the vagina. Vaginal stricture, a narrowing of the vagina, and a shortened vagina, later causing painful intercourse, were two other results of the surgery. Beyond these developments, however, there are often longer-range repercussions. Even after a "successful" hysterectomy, these repercussions may include reduced sex drive, weight gain, and depression. A woman should know that these possibilities exist and should assess their impact carefully, so that after surgery she can recover and continue productively with her life.

Psychological Impact of Hysterectomy

Women who have had hysterectomies that were clearly lifesaving procedures, as with cancer, tend to feel less doubt about whether or not the operation was necessary. This is understandable. However, there is a thread of doubt that may haunt some women whose hysterectomies were not performed as a lifesaving measure. For them, the removal of the uterus (and ovaries) during their reproductive years, or even premature to natural menopause, may cause profound feelings of inadequacy. These feelings are connected to the loss of the physical sources of femininity—the reproductive organs—and the result may be anger, depression, sadness, and lack of self-esteem.

Most of these feelings tend to surface about three months or longer after surgery, when the body has had time to heal. Depression related to a "loss of femininity," the fear of becoming androgynous from lack of ovarian hormones, and the fear of growing unattractive to her mate can greatly affect the realities of the woman's life. Many women, however, come to view their hysterectomy as a psychological and physiological challenge. Granted, this can be a more wrenching process for a young woman given an unnecessary hysterectomy.

In my own practice, each woman who has had a hysterectomy has found her own way to resume a normal life—and even to improve it in many cases. My suggestion is for you to speak to others who have had the surgery and to try to understand everything about what may happen. Then, for your own peace of mind *postoperatively,* you will need to confront the range of feelings, good and bad (there may be relief from pain and bleeding, along with ambivalence about the surgery). Counseling may help you sort out the realities of hysterectomy in terms of your sexuality and femininity.

POSSIBLE AFTEREFFECTS OF HYSTERECTOMY

• *Psychosexual:* Hysterectomy can usher in a wide range of emotional responses involving altered feelings about femininity, body image, and the fear of becoming unattractive to one's mate. Not every hysterectomy patient suffers from such a negative aftermath, but many women do need to take steps to ward off depression, a sense of inadequacy, anger, and guilt, and to maintain a healthy and realistic sense of being a woman.

One effect of ovarian and uterine loss is reduced sex drive, primarily related to the elimination of ovarian hormones, including ovarian androgens, hormones directly linked to sexual interest. But the loss of these hormones alone is not entirely responsible for diminished sexuality. Studies indicate that the uterus, like the clitoris and vagina, becomes engorged with blood during the excitement phase of sexual arousal and contributes to increased sexual pleasure.

Any woman whose sex drive has been impaired by hysterectomy must—to put it bluntly—fight back! I suggest that she start by improving her general health, following the vitamin and nutritional guidelines mapped out in this book. To revitalize body tissue and work to restore her prehysterectomy libido, she will need to begin a carefully prescribed hormone replacement program. A number of studies indicate that a combination of androgen and estrogen may help restore libido physiologically. Other women may respond favorably to hormone replacement therapy (HRT). Estrogen-content vaginal creams can increase blood supply to the vagina and maintain its sensitivity.

• *Hot flashes:* Of all symptoms of menopause and hysterectomy, none is so well known as this sudden surge of heat that visibly radiates from the upper torso to the face. Hot flashes affect up to 50 percent of women who have had hysterectomies, and up to 85 percent of women who have gone through natural menopause. Lasting about two or three minutes on the average, hot flashes bring with them

209

dizziness, heart palpitations, sweating, and deep flushes to the face. While they are not health-threatening, hot flashes cause discomfort and may disrupt sleep. Science has yet to pinpoint the actual cause of these flashes, but it has been found that stimulants such as coffee, alcohol, and nicotine can aggravate the problem.

• *Osteoporosis:* Osteoporosis is a progressive thinning of the bones that affects about 25 percent of postmenopausal women, who may lose up to 30 percent of their bone mass. Osteoporosis can increase the chances of bone fracture, bone fragility, the deterioration of the spine and hip joints, and the development of a "dowager's hump." Complications of osteoporosis can even lead to death in some cases. Estrogen is directly related to bone density and bone rebuilding, since it stimulates the life-giving supply of calcium to bone tissue. After menopause, estrogen levels drop, and you may be at risk for this serious disorder. While it is a serious condition for women going through a natural menopause, the risk of osteoporosis can be even greater for women who undergo surgical menopause, via hysterectomy. Natural menopause can create a slower, though steady, loss of bone over time. The suddenness of surgically produced menopause produces an estrogen withdrawal in the extreme.

Estrogen replacement (ERT) is especially recommended for women who show a family history of osteoporosis, who tend toward bone fractures, or who have calcium deficiencies. (Be aware of what is involved in ERT—see below.) Foods rich in calcium are recommended on a daily basis (tofu, dairy products, calcium-enriched cereals and pastas, broccoli and spinach) supplemented with calcium in tablet form, such as 2,500 mg of calcium taken with 400 units of vitamin D. Weight-bearing exercise has been shown to *increase* bone mass, so I would also recommend a program of exercise, such as low-impact aerobics or walking.

• *Vaginal atrophy:* This condition brings to mind apprehensive visions of withering—but they are visions far beyond the actual picture. Lowered levels of estrogen can cause a thinning and drying of the cells lining the vagina.

This results in a loss of muscle tone of the vaginal walls and itchiness and a burning sensation due to diminished natural lubrication. Intercourse can be irritating and painful. Vaginal atrophy may not be evident until months or years following hysterectomy, depending on the woman. The only way to restore the vagina to its normal resiliency is with hormone replacement (HRT); it is the answer for any woman who intends to be sexually active.

• *Risk of cardiovascular disease:* Most recent studies indicate that estrogen may be instrumental in preventing the onset of cardiovascular disorders. The chances of heart attack, hardening of the arteries (ateriosclerosis), and high blood pressure (which can lead to stroke) are increased among women who have had hysterectomies.

WHAT HORMONES ARE NECESSARY AFTER HYSTERECTOMY?

After a total abdominal hysterectomy with removal of the ovaries, hormone replacement therapy (HRT) will eventually be called for. HRT involves supplements combining doses of estrogen and progestin; ERT (estrogen replacement therapy) is the use of estrogen alone.

In determining which hormone replacement system is best for you, we would need to evaluate the many studies being done on this very question. Growing evidence seems to indicate that the balance of estrogen and progesterone in hormone replacement therapy (HRT) is the safest mode of estrogen replacement. One reason is an apparently decreased risk of cancer when estrogen is combined with progesterone. Cancers of the reproductive system have been associated with estrogen treatment given alone. Progesterone has the ability to keep estrogen in check, working with estrogen to mimic the body's natural hormone balance.

When it first was made available, estrogen replacement appeared to be the medical miracle that menopausal women had long been waiting for. Estrogen replacement, however, evolved into a complicated matter, and one early development of ERT was its abuse. Doctors who did not understand the eventual effects of estrogen supplements on the body prescribed high doses of the drug over long periods of time without a break. The consequences of such imprudent use of ERT soon became evident among women who did not have hysterectomies: reports of endometrial cancer were apparently related to this high-dosage estrogen therapy. In fact, it was found that estrogen replacement alone increased the risks of uterine cancer in many women by up to ten times, no doubt a result of estrogen's inherent ability to trigger the growth of the uterine lining.

More recent studies have investigated the link, if any, between ERT and breast cancer, but thus far, the evidence is inconclusive. Clearly, if you have had a hysterectomy, you will not have to worry about the possibility of being at risk for developing uterine cancer. Women with hysterectomies, however, should be on estrogen replacement only for a short time, since overstimulation of estrogen alone could enhance the possibilities of breast cancer. If they plan on long-term hormone replacement, it may be wiser to choose the progesterone–estrogen formula.

Estrogen replacement therapy has become more refined in the last decade as scientists have come to understand the nuances of hormones in the body—both in menopausal women with low levels of ovarian hormones and those who have had hysterectomies including ovarian removal. There now exist many different options for estrogen and estrogen–progesterone therapies following hysterectomy. Which one you choose will be an individual matter decided upon with your doctor's guidance. Here is an overview of what is available and what it can do for you:

Often, *natural* ovarian estrogens are used for ERT, rather than the synthetic estrogens that are normally found in birth control pills. The dosage required for estrogen replacement is much lower than is needed for contraceptive measures. This dosage is thought sufficient to prevent cardiovascular problems, such as increased risk of heart attack and high blood pressure, as well as irreversible osteoporosis. Women taking the .6-mg pill who still have disruptive menopausal symptoms, such as hot flashes, may need a slightly higher dosage.

Premarin, the most often-consumed estrogen replacement product, has been in use for approximately forty years. Other estrogens in pill form used for ERT are Ogen, Estratab, and Estrace. They range in strength of dosage, but they are all prescribed for a regimen of one pill a day for either twenty-one or twenty-five days a month. ERT may also be taken in the form of vaginal creams, such as Premarin, Ogen, Estraguard, and Ortho Dienestrol. The most up-to-date approach to ERT is with Estraderm (estradiol transdermal system), an "estrogen patch" which delivers a low-dosage natural estrogen through the skin at a constant rate—a time-release formula, so to speak. A round patch with adhesive borders, Estraderm allows the direct absorption of estrogen into the bloodstream. Hormone pills, in contrast, must travel through the gastrointestinal tract and to the liver, where the estrogen is broken down chemically and finally secreted into the blood. The quantity of estrogen in pill form is higher than that found in patches; this higher amount allows for what will remain usable after breakdown in the liver. Each standard patch contains only .05 mg of estrogen and two such patches must be used consecutively each week to absorb the right dosage.

Hormone replacement therapy (HRT) can employ a similar course of treatment with the identical estrogen products, but with the addition of progesterone. HRT works most effectively when estrogen (such as Premarin) is given alone from days one through fourteen. This is followed by estrogen and progesterone for the next seven to ten days of either 10 mg of Provera or 5 mg of Aygestin. No hormones are given for the next five to seven days.

Women will need hormone supplements following hysterectomy, but I do not recommend them for six months to a year after surgery for complications of endometriosis. During this time without estrogen, any residual endometriosis can "burn itself out." If HRT or ERT is given too soon after surgery, it will keep alive any microscopic endometriosis that may be located, for example, on the bowel or the bladder. I recommend that a woman first take Danocrine for at least three months for these reasons:

• It can melt away any vestiges of endometriosis.

• It will help offset the symptoms of sudden estrogen withdrawal (such as hot flashes) due to removal of the ovaries.

• It will not interfere with proper calcium absorption or deplete bone tissue and cause osteoporosis.

By the end of three months (or six months in severe cases), any remaining endometriosis tissue should have disappeared. A few months after the termination of Danocrine, there should be no spontaneous recurrence of the disease.

About twelve months after surgery, ERT or HRT may be initiated. The type of hormone supplement will depend on what the doctor feels is the best choice for his patient. If a woman on estrogen replacement therapy begins to experience pelvic pain, cramps, or severe abdominal pain that feels like earlier endometriosis symptoms, she should contact her doctor immediately. He will determine if endometriosis has recurred and whether or not she should be taken off this hormone therapy.

HOLD ON TO YOUR ORGANS

It is because of the possible long-range effects that I urge women to understand the procedures involved in hysterectomies and not to give their doctors permission to perform this surgery except in the most urgent cases. When women go in for a simple removal of ovarian cysts and are given complete hysterectomies, with removal of uterus, ovaries, and tubes, this is not only unnecessary but wrong.

Although it is impossible to generalize about hysterectomy, when questioned, many women who have had this surgery feel relieved to know that the source of pain or disease has been removed, but they also suffer emotional loss. Women often worry that their hysterectomy was unnecessary, especially if it was performed during their reproductive years. Removing the ovaries of a young and previously fertile woman stops hormone production, and she is, in essence, castrated.

The uterus is more than an internal "baby buggy." It is an endocrinologically *active* organ, "the cradle of creativity" to many women and thus worthy of lifelong care.

In my practice I have treated several hundred women over the last ten years who were told that total hysterectomy was the obvious answer to their problems with endometriosis. In all these "hopeless" cases, I did a careful examination and evaluation to determine the exact problem. In each case, I advised these women against hysterectomy and successfully treated them so that they now have much improved lives.

One case especially impressed me. Renee, who is thirty-two years old, traveled from Philadelphia for a consultation with me. Renee told me that she had been suffering from pelvic pain for nine years. During this time, she had seen six different doctors. They had prescribed drugs ranging from antibiotics to Demerol to morphine without Renee's showing any improvement. She and her husband had given up on having a child, and when the opportunity had presented itself, they adopted a girl. Three different doctors had suggested hysterectomy. The idea of this surgery horrified her, but she didn't see how she could avoid it. Her mother-in-law finally pressed Renee to get a *seventh* opinion—this was how I met her.

Renee was clearly a victim of endometriosis that had not been treated properly. After a physical examination and lengthy talk with her, I told Renee that she did not need a hysterectomy. I was sure her condition would be helped through a change in diet and vitamin intake, modified exercise, and Danocrine. Thus began Renee's regimen to eliminate the disease.

Although she was able to tolerate Danocrine, Renee began to develop increased abdominal pain after four months on the drug. I scheduled her for a laparoscopy, during which I removed many of her pelvic and tubal adhesions and other remnants of the disease on other pelvic organs.

Renee continued on Danocrine for three months following surgery. I recommended that if she wanted a child, she should try and get pregnant immediately after stopping Danocrine. She had been told by other doctors that she needed fertility drugs, but I felt her physical condition was so improved and her outlook on life so completely changed that she could try to conceive without them. When she came for a follow-up visit two months after discontinuing Danocrine, she complained of feeling worse than she had four months before. She was afraid that the endometriosis had come back. Careful examination revealed no sign of the disease; rather, to her pleasure and mine, Renee's urine pregnancy test came out positive!

Renee took exceptional care of herself during pregnancy, and she had one of the easiest deliveries that I have ever seen. She conceived again the following year, and she now has another son. It goes without saying that Renee is thankful that her mother-in-law insisted on a seventh opinion.

WHAT YOU SHOULD KNOW ABOUT EXPLORATORY SURGERY

One way to avoid unnecessary hysterectomy may be through meticulously carried out exploratory surgery, and Renee's case is a perfect example of this. During an exploratory, the doctor can do his best to save organs and clean away much of the endometriosis.

"Will this surgery actually help my endometriosis or will it just add to my problems?" patients ask when I advise an exploratory. Others tell me: "I fear a hysterectomy. Please tell me what can be done to prevent it."

The prospect of surgery can cause great anxiety, especially when the exact nature of an abdominal mass is unknown, but endometriosis is suspected. One reason for conservative, or exploratory, surgery is for the doctor to determine the extent of abdominal endometriosis and to remove some of the larger cysts. A woman with severe endometriosis who has not been helped by Danocrine alone may be the perfect candidate for exploratory surgery. This is surgery designed to excise endometrial cysts, clear up adhesions where possible, and repair organs rather than remove them.

If the doctor suspects that his patient has a large ovarian endometriotic cyst, for example, or a pelvic mass that he believes is caused by endometriosis, a sonogram can help confirm if the pelvic abnormality is endometriosis. If it is, the doctor should prescribe Danocrine prior to surgery to reduce or eliminate the endometrial masses and decrease formation of new adhesions. I suggest a dosage of 200 mg three times a day for at least three months before entering the hospital. This drug treatment makes surgery easier: Danocrine shrinks endometriotic tissue, making what remains less bloody when it is surgically excised. This simple drug treatment prior to surgery can prevent hysterectomy in many cases.

After the Danocrine program, surgery to remove an ovarian cyst, for example, can then be performed. It is best done through a Pfannenstiel, or bikini-line, incision—a cut below the upper edge of the pubic hairline. The scar formed from a fine Pfannenstiel incision eventually will be hidden by pubic hair or fade completely. The doctor will then explore the pelvic organs. If an ovarian cyst is present, he can gently remove it without damaging or removing the ovary. This is a critical point in surgery: the doctor must think about the woman's future and do what he can to preserve her organs.

After removal of a cyst, the ovaries can be repaired with microsurgical techniques. Then the doctor will "lyse" adhesions, that is, free organs that are stuck together, between the bowel and other organs, for example, a common site for them to grow. Freeing, or lysis, of adhesions usually results in less pelvic pain and is a practical surgical decision. It is often the pulling motion between the bowel and fibrous adhesions that causes cramping and pain each time there is a peristaltic or bowel movement.

Next, if the uterus is tilted backward, a uterine suspension may be performed using a technique called a modified Gilliam's suspension. Here the round ligaments that hold the uterus in position are pulled up and shortened, thereby moving the uterus forward and preventing it from dropping backward again. This procedure places the organs in their normal position, increasing the chances of conception.

After surgery is completed, and before the abdominal cavity is closed, all measures to prevent adhesions should be scrupulously taken (what these measures entail will be explained shortly). Since adhesions cause such pain for sufferers of endometriosis, this is a critical step in surgery.

PREPARING YOURSELF FOR SURGERY

Unless there is good cause for more immediate surgery, such as uncontrollable bleeding, your doctor will tell you that you have a few weeks to a few months before you are admitted to the hospital. Use this time to prepare for the surgery.

• *Strengthen your immune system* by increasing your dosage of vitamin supplements. Take 500 mg of vitamin C twice a day, 50 mg of zinc three times a day, 400 IU of vitamin E twice a day, 10,000 IU of beta-carotene once a day, 40 mg of iron once a day (to increase your blood count), and 100 mg of B complex (to help reduce stress).

• *Watch your diet* and cut down on fat, salt, and sugar. If you tend to be overweight or to gain weight in the midsection, try to lose weight. Less fatty tissue in the abdominal area makes surgery easier and ensures less chance of infection.

• *Take light exercise* before surgery to strengthen your cardiovascular system. A fifteen-minute to half-hour walk at a steady pace will oxygenate your system and keep muscles toned.

How Can the Doctor Prevent Adhesions During Surgery?

"I don't fear surgery as much as I fear adhesions," a young woman told me. "The two operations I had to remove ovarian cysts resulted in terrible adhesions, especially covering one tube. Isn't there a way to prevent these growths?"

Adhesion formation after surgery can create its own breed of pelvic problems, such as growing around fallopian tubes and ovaries and binding them together. Happily, many standard techniques that can help prevent or greatly lessen the chances of adhesions are now available to surgeons. Actual elimination of these fibrous growths may begin with the surgeon himself—that is, he must not only be skillful but should work smoothly, efficiently, and knowledgeably. Sloppy doctors can be instrumental in undoing their good surgical work by not being meticulous with the details.

During surgery, bleeding areas must be tied off or cauterized. The

217

risk of adhesions will increase if the doctor leaves bloody or oozing surfaces after closing an incision. The finest suture, or surgical fiber, should be used (as if for delicate microsurgery), not the heavier, more irritating catgut. Finally, a high-molecular, viscous, and slightly greasy solution, Dextran-70 or Hyskon, can be placed in the abdomen before closing it. This substance coats organs and ensures that they move smoothly against each other rather than stick together to form new adhesions.

Medication can make recovery faster and simpler, too. Hydrocortisone, a known anti-inflammatory drug, can help during and after surgery. Before closing the incision, 200 mg of hydrocortisone can be mixed with Dextran-70 and placed in the abdomen. Following surgery, I prescribe for my patients 100 mg of hydrocortisone every six hours for the first twenty-four hours, followed by 100 mg every eight hours for the next twenty-four hours, and 100 mg every twelve hours on the third day. This three-day course in combination with intravenous antibiotics has been proved to cut down on adhesions. An anti-inflammatory medication, such as Motrin, in a dosage of 600–800 mg given four times daily over two weeks following surgery also cuts down on these fibrous growths.

Using this surgical program to prevent adhesions is most often a successful procedure, and protects a woman from adhesions in the event of future surgery. I have discovered that if my patients require surgery in the future, such as for cesarean sections, there is rarely any formation of adhesions as a result of a prior operation when it is done in the manner just described.

ARE THERE OTHER SURGICAL OPTIONS FOR ENDOMETRIOSIS?

There are a few surgical treatments for endometriosis that were common at one time. In my opinion, two in particular are dated and not as consistently beneficial as they might be. Some doctors, in trying to avoid hysterectomy, attempt to help their patients either by doing a *presacral neurectomy* or an appendectomy. I recently corresponded with a twenty-seven-year-old restaurant manager in Michigan who brought up this exact dilemma.

Marjorie confessed that she keeps delaying her upcoming operation, out of doubt. She wrote candidly: "I've always had very bad menstrual cramps, so it's just a fact of life to me. But in the last four years, I've been getting terrible backaches and pain shooting down my legs. Since I'm on my feet so much at the restaurant, I can barely get through the day without wanting to scream. The doctor gave me codeine, but it stopped working for me a long time ago.

"I went back to him a month ago because I thought I was having an appendicitis attack—that's how bad the pain was on my right side. The doctor told me that I have a large ovarian cyst on my right ovary, caused by endometriosis. He wants to operate and take out the cyst, as well as my appendix, which he says I don't need and which the endometriosis might affect to the point where it would rupture. For the back pain, he told me that a presacral neurectomy might be the only answer. I don't want a hysterectomy at my age, but my doctor has suggested it. I'm worried that I'll go in for an appendectomy and come out without my uterus. Please help me."

Marjorie's plight is not an uncommon one. Women with pain in their right sides may be diagnosed as having appendicitis, and a great number of them undergo unnecessary appendectomies because of a confusion of symptoms. Every sharp and persistent pain on the right side does not mean that the appendix is involved. An actual appendicitis attack is accompanied by symptoms of nausea and vomiting, usually for several days prior to the "attack," as well as diarrhea and fever. If there is only pain, it may be, for example, a ruptured ovarian cyst or hormonal fluctuations affecting endometriotic tissue.

When the cyst is larger and troublesome, as in Marjorie's case, I believe surgery would eventually be the answer. But first a regimen of three months of Danocrine should be administered. This might shrink the cyst and perhaps eliminate the need for surgery. If there is still pain, Marjorie may only need a laparoscopy to examine the pelvic organs. Should the cyst be evident during this procedure, exploratory surgery would be necessary to remove the cyst, but not the ovary. If her doctor insists *before surgery* that he will remove the ovary, which still has healthy tissue, she should find a doctor who is willing to preserve her organs. Removing the appendix is not indicated for endometriosis and is rarely done today. In one study, doctors found only two cases among fifty-six patients where endometriosis affected the appendix. It is worth noting that in these cases, endometriosis was not the cause of the appendicitis.

It is also my feeling that the appendix has an important function in immune system strengthening and regulation, and this taken-for-granted organ may even be somehow linked to cancer prevention. This small abdominal organ is filled with lymphatic tissue, known for its antibody formation. Antibodies are necessary factors in destroying invading bacteria and cancer cells.

219

A presacral neurectomy, also advised for Marjorie, is complicated because it involves cutting nerve tissue. A relatively difficult procedure, presacral neurectomy may also be done during exploratory surgery, taking in all about thirty to forty minutes. For the last twenty years or so, this type of surgery was recommended for women with extreme dysmenorrhea (painful menstruation) or to increase chances of conception.

A presacral neurectomy involves surgery on an area behind the uterus and in front of the spine where all the nerves enter into the pelvic area and the legs. The presacral nerve contains nerve tissue that influences the contractions of the uterus and fallopian tubes. Since uterine contractions from prostaglandins can cause infertility, doctors believed that by cutting the nerve, they were also cutting down on uterine hyperactivity.

Some women have been pleased with the results of this surgery, finding that they are greatly improved. A number of doctors report that a greater percentage of their infertile patients have become pregnant following a presacral neurectomy. Others, however, showed no discrepancy in conception rates with or without such an operation, and most doctors don't recommend it today. A presacral neurectomy also carries with it the danger of cutting other key nerves, which later can cause difficulty in controlling bladder or bowel functions.

I think that such surgery would not be Marjorie's best course of action, since there are other, more effective alternatives to her problem of painful menstruation. I personally have performed very few presacral neurectomies, much preferring the safer resectioning and shortening of the uterosacral ligaments that stretch up behind the uterus. In this procedure, a quarter of an inch of ligament is cut off, thereby also cutting some of the main nerve endings. The two ends are then sewn together, suspending the uterus at the same time. This places the uterus in a more normal, upright position, increasing chances of conception. When the uterus is thus lifted away from irritating prostaglandin secretions in the peritoneal cavity, patients may also note a greater decrease in pain.

Doctors can also aid in decreasing back and uterine pain by coagulating or burning off a portion of the uterosacral ligament during laparoscopy rather than during exploratory surgery. This can only be done when there are no extensive masses of adhesions pulling the uterus back, making it difficult to identify the uterosacral ligament itself. If her doctor opts for this procedure, along with uterine suspension if it is called for, Marjorie is more likely to have a pain-free recovery and keep her organs.

UTERINE FIBROIDS AND ENDOMETRIOSIS

Not every woman with uterine fibroids also suffers from endometriosis, and not every woman struggling with endometriosis shows any signs of fibroids. However, both conditions often do coexist, and they have many patterns of growth in common. "If fibroids can cause uterine bleeding, won't I need a hysterectomy to clear up both problems at once?" patients ask. It's a good question. Both conditions are complex, but they often can be resolved successfully.

A fibroid, like endometriosis, may be microscopic or extremely large in size, but oddly enough, fibroids can go undetected. *Unlike* many endometrial cysts, large or small, the presence of fibroids is less often signaled by pain, cramps, or bleeding. As common as they are, about 99 percent of all fibroid tumors, also called myomas or leimyomas, are noncancerous and are the primary reason for an enlarged uterus.

How do you know if you have fibroids? A competent physician can usually detect the presence of a tumor and gauge its size and location during a routine pelvic examination. If there is any confusion about the location of the tumor (sometimes a doctor cannot tell if the tumor is uterine or ovarian), a sonogram or laparoscopy should reveal its precise nature. However, one type of fibroid, called a submucous fibroid, lies between uterine walls and tends to distort the uterine cavity. To verify its type, doctors may perform a hysterosalpingogram, or X ray of the uterus and tubes, if a sonogram first fails to produce conclusive evidence.

How common are fibroids? About one in five women over thirty years of age is thought to have this uterine problem. Black women tend to develop them five times more frequently, and Eastern European and Jewish women are known to be more susceptible to fibroids, too. Very few prepubescent girls or postmenopausal women develop these tumors; the growth of fibroids remains, like endometriosis, linked to estrogen levels and the reproductive years. Fibroids are known to enlarge rapidly when a woman is pregnant and her estrogen levels are highest. Estrogen-containing birth control pills are also responsible for causing these normally slow-growing tumors to flourish. Obese women are warned to have their doctors monitor their fibroids, since a high percentage of body fat stimulates estrogen production.

Several theories exist as to why these uterine tumors develop. Heredity appears to be the one consistent point between them, although other discrepancies arise. In fact, family predisposition is one of the

221

strongest factors in predicting the development of these myomas. Some scientists believe that a woman may be born with the *seed* of it in the uterine wall. This theory is similar to the embryonic theory of endometriosis. But why a fibroid grows still remains an unknown, although it definitely is linked to female hormone production.

In researching how fibroids develop, scientists have examined all aspects of the myoma and its growth patterns. One theory of their origin is based on visible evidence: microscopic examination of fibroids reveal that they are largely composed of muscle cells. Therefore, these theorists hold, myomas develop from the smooth muscle cells of the uterine wall. Another theory is that these tumors arise from fibrous or connective cells, not muscle tissue cells, of the uterine wall. A third theory is based on the idea of abnormal cell development; that is, fibroids occur when the developing muscle cells, fibrous cells, or blood vessels do not grow normally into their respective organs and, instead, form tumors.

Types of Fibroids and How to Treat Them

The type of fibroid you have, and how many, will determine whether or not giveaway clues will reveal their presence. This accounts for the surprise many women feel when they are examined for one problem and the doctor discovers fibroids. First, there is the typically pain-free myoma, or the intramural or interstitial fibroid, most often located in the middle of the muscular wall of the uterus. The intramural fibroid usually causes no pain when it is small, but larger ones can occasionally obstruct the vagina during childbirth. The subserous, or subperitoneal, fibroids grow anywhere on the outside of the uterus, sandwiched beneath the peritoneum or the outer lining of the uterus. Subserous myomas may be painful, but paradoxically, they can become large and cause no pain at all. When they are located in front of the uterus, they may press on the bladder, creating difficult or frequent urination. Growing on the lower part of the uterus, the subserous tumor can make vaginal delivery impossible if the growth is large enough to block the vagina. Subserous fibroids tend to bleed more frequently than the intramural variety.

When a subserous fibroid grows into a mushroom shape, with a stalklike protuberance attached to the uterine wall, it is called a pedunculated myoma. The pedunculated fibroid is less problematic unless it twists around its own stalk. When this happens, the blood supply to the tumor is cut off, causing extreme pain.

A third type of fibroid that may be known to women with endometriosis is the submucous fibroid: it is the least common of the three types, but the most troublesome. Submucous fibroids protrude into the uterine cavity—only growing inside the uterine wall—where they can enlarge, tear uterine lining, and set off a bout of heavy bleeding. Pregnancy can be difficult when these tumors exist, disturbing the normal growth and blood supply of the placenta, and sometimes causing miscarriage. Submucous fibroids also pedunculate; however, since they are located in the uterus, the body responds to them as if they were foreign objects and tries to expel them through contractions. Occasionally, the force of uterine contractions will push the fibroid through the cervix while the stalk is stubbornly attached to the uterine wall.

If you have fibroids, you should have checkups twice a year to monitor their size and growth rates. Though it is not always the case, rapid growth can indicate malignancy. Except for the natural cure—menopause—or pseudomenopause engendered by drugs like the new agonists or Danocrine, there is no known cure for fibroids.

Troublesome fibroids that cause you chronic pain or bleeding are best treated by surgery. The operation, called a myomectomy, is an attempt to remove all visible fibroids, thereby saving the uterus and avoiding hysterectomy. Doctors may use electrocautery, the scalpel, or laser surgery to remove them. Afterward, sutures of microsurgical quality, which create fine closures, are used to repair the uterus, restoring it to as normal an appearance as is possible. I have performed hundreds of these operations, and found that they can be very successful and almost bloodless procedures. The point is to preserve the uterus, permitting future childbearing if a woman so chooses. A woman with damaged fallopian tubes due to endometriosis who is also suffering from uterine fibroids may benefit from a myomectomy. If she does not conceive naturally, she could increase her chances of bearing a child using the newer *in vitro* fertilization techniques discussed in the previous chapter.

Surgery may not be necessary for some fibroids. If a woman has a combination of fibroids and endometriosis, she will doubly benefit from Danocrine, which is known to shrink fibroids up to 50 percent. I'd suggest 600 mg a day for three to six months. This drug therapy might completely eliminate the endometriosis and shrink fibroids to such an extent that a woman becomes symptom-free. If the fibroid uterus is less than the size of a three-month pregnancy and there are no symptoms, no further treatment is necessary. Be sure to keep your weight down, since weight gain increases estrogen, which will spur the growth of fibroids. If you wish to have a baby, the few months following surgery and Danocrine treatment would be a good time to try to conceive.

If a woman still has pain from fibroids, and they are causing her uterus to be larger than the size of a three-month pregnancy, I would recommend exploratory surgery to perform a myomectomy, lysis of pelvic adhesions, electrocautery or laser surgery of all visible endo- metriosis lesions, and, if it is called for, a uterine suspension. This surgery should be followed by Danocrine for three to six months to shrink microscopic endometrial implants and remaining fibroids.

In cases of adenomyosis (endometriosis interna) in combination with fibroids, the same treatment courses should be taken, but the chance of avoiding hysterectomy is slimmer—particularly if ade- nomyosis is extensive. Remember, adenomyosis tissue involves the entire uterine wall, and these growths cannot be removed one by one, as with fibroids. Adenomyosis can so damage the uterus that there is continuous bleeding, and hysterectomy may be the only answer. I urge women to see an endometriosis specialist and to be treated with an endometriosis drug alone or in combination with a myomectomy. This regimen has, in my own experience, proved very beneficial, improving the general well-being of many, many women, as well as providing new opportunities for successful pregnancies and childbear- ing.

Is a Hysterectomy Advised if an Endometriotic Cyst Is Cancerous?

Although it is a rarity, endometriosis cells have the potential of becoming cancerous. Unfortunately, very few warning signs precede it. Because the "hidden disease" can grow into malignancy, sufferers of endometriosis should be sure to have follow-up visits with their doctors every six months. Each time, the doctor can determine if there are any new pelvic masses, as well as check on the size of existing cysts. A sonogram might be indicated to determine the nature of any suspicious mass, followed by laparoscopy or exploratory surgery. During either of these surgical procedures, a sample of tissue can be taken and biopsied for malignancy.

It is important that women with persistent ovarian cysts be tested to see if the cyst is benign. If it is malignant, there is little chance of avoiding a hysterectomy, unless the cancer is *in situ* or just starting to develop. In that case, the doctor can remove one ovary and not the other. However, with ovarian cancer, the chance of it developing and spreading to the other ovary is very high. Then a total hysterectomy is indicated. After surgery, an oncologist, or cancer specialist, will evaluate the cancer and most likely recommend chemotherapy.

Such endometriosis is rare, but it is important that you realize that such potential exists. In most cases, endometriosis can be cured or greatly improved with conservative surgery and medication so you can live normally, keep your organs, and still conceive if you care to. Take the opportunity to work with a good endometriosis specialist who can best treat you in the way you deserve.

If it happens that a hysterectomy is indicated for your case, you should know exactly what is involved in the surgical process and what to expect during recovery and beyond.

TRY TO SAY NO TO HYSTERECTOMY

Hysterectomy is not a cure for endometriosis.

If all avenues have been explored—Danocrine therapy, the endometriosis diet, vitamins, laser surgery, or any of the alternate treatments to alleviate pain, like acupuncture—and you are still in extreme pain, try each program another time around. You will always do best to preserve your organs as long as you can. Remember, removal of the reproductive organs does not guarantee that all the endometriosis has been eliminated.

If you get two or three opinions about your endometriosis and are told that you have extreme adhesions and other pelvic complications demanding a hysterectomy, insist on surgery where you can keep at least one ovary. Do not allow your age to influence the decision. Women thirty-six years and older are most commonly counseled to have a hysterectomy. The thinking is that they are premenopausal, so there is no harm in trimming back their reproductive years. Such thinking cheats you and it does not help your condition, since hormone replacement therapy (HRT) can usher in a new bout of the disease.

In view of the great achievements in research today, I urge women to take a very conservative stand on hysterectomy. The better cure may be just around the corner.

CHAPTER 14

There Is Hope

WOMEN have made considerable gains in their lives over the last few decades, and I think the most considerable of all is their passionate interest in—and pursuit of—optimal health. Every woman in America has access to information that may help her understand her body and what is happening to it. What she reads may save her life. As a doctor, I know this is true. A book or magazine article or professional journal can clarify a previously misdiagnosed medical problem, or, in fact, bring a condition to a woman's attention, spurring her to seek immediate medical advice.

As I see it, the willingness to be in tune with her body gives the contemporary woman a greater chance for a better and longer life, free of endometriosis. This book is designed to provide some of the knowledge that would make the goal of a healthier life possible.

We have progressed beyond the days when disease was thought of as an invincible force one was powerless to fight. As I mentioned early in this book, it has been outdated *attitudes* about being female, and myths about the female body, that can create, in very real ways, serious health threats to women.

Confusion about the identification and treatment of endometriosis is no longer as common an occurrence. Fewer doctors view endometriosis with tunnel vision—no longer dismissing it as a menstrually related problem that can be "cured" only by a hysterectomy. Doctors have expanded their attention to the disease as well as their knowledge and understanding of it. There is more research than ever exploring the intricacies of the disease. Endometriosis will never again be a complicated secret, ravaging a woman's life. Because of the insidious nature of endometriosis, some confusion still exists, *but there can be an end to this if women speak up.*

This book supplies the facts about the disease. It tells how other women have felt about and coped with it, sometimes over a lifetime, and it reveals the newest, most effective treatments in ending the misery of endometriosis. I have lectured all over the United States and I always stress to women that health care must begin with themselves. I fervently believe this. If they are vigilant in monitoring the course of the disease, and get past all the barriers that might prevent them from seeking a specialist (such as fear or shyness), they cannot help but improve.

It is my hope that every woman reading these pages will *be set on a course of action that can help her conquer endometriosis.* This disease continues to afflict millions of working women. Endometriosis coexists with stress-filled lives; it grows as immune systems falter and endurance is pushed to the limit. It may spread when childbearing is delayed. It can strike, and strike again, many high-risk candidates: those working women who also have a strong family predisposition to the disease. Every woman has the right to shape her own life—either to view marriage and motherhood as her career, to combine family care and work in a personally devised formula that suits her, or to forfeit motherhood and devote herself entirely to achievement, or any variation therein. She is entitled to be free of endometriosis to enjoy the life she has chosen.

In this book, I have examined a number of pathways that the woman with endometriosis can follow. Because the disease will vary so widely, cure involves a number of crucial steps.

• *Be attuned to early symptoms.* Earliest awareness makes prevention and cure easier. This "triad" of symptoms often occurs together and signals the possibility of endometriosis: menstrual cramps, painful intercourse, and infertility. It is my feeling that the early telling symptoms of endometriosis should be clear to you and to your doctor. If he is an expert, he may not need to do a laparoscopy to verify his diagnosis, even if there were no clinical symptoms of minimal endometriosis during a physical examination.

• *Be aware of treatments that are right for you if your case is mild.* Not all endometriosis needs drug therapy or surgical intervention. You can often administer some of the best medicine by changing your life-style and dietary patterns. Actual physiological changes—detrimental or beneficial—are triggered by certain foods, vitamins, exercise, stress, and mood.

I have detailed this for you in chapter 9. In brief, I suggest an increase of B vitamins, calcium, and magnesium; a decrease in fats (which stimulate unwanted estrogen production and the growth of endometriotic tissue); a cutback on dairy foods and fruit, which have been shown to be somewhat of a factor in irritating endometriosis; and a reduction in salt, sugar, and junk food intake to keep weight stabilized.

Add to these dietary helpmates an increase of exercise, de-stressing programs, alternate treatments to relieve pain, such as acupuncture, or over-the-counter prostaglandin inhibitors (such as ibuprofen, Advil, and Motrin).

Microscopic endometriosis can be halted in the earliest stages with low-estrogen birth control pills. This treatment is best for young women or those who are at high risk for developing the disease. Remember, however, that birth control pills *should never be given* to the woman with verified endometriosis, diagnosed even in its earliest stage, or to any woman who has had surgery for the disease. Women who have had endometriosis verified, no matter how mild the case, especially if they do not wish to conceive right away, may benefit from a three-to-six-month treatment using Danocrine to shrink away the endometriosis tissue.

• *Be alert to treatments and health care if your case is more severe.* Although drug therapy and surgery to remove the larger lesions will help, I must reemphasize the need for good nutrition and exercise in these cases. More severe endometriosis demands more attention and greater effort to cure. I have had many successes in treating women, using a carefully monitored combination of diet, drug therapy, and, if required, exploratory or laser surgery to excise as much of the disease as is possible. Danocrine, or one of the other analogs that will be available in the near future, effectively shrinks endometriosis as well as reduces the size of uterine fibroids and adenomyosis.

• *Be aware of your options.* Because there is no one answer to curing endometriosis, I have included every approach a specialist in this disease might advise for a patient. What may work for one woman may be a marginal answer to another, especially when we are dealing with drugs. Toleration levels differ. However, certain of the newer surgical techniques like videolaseroscopy in the hands of an expert can change nearly every sufferer's life for the better. This is one procedure that can offer relief or cure because of its precise excision of lesions, even those the size of a pinhead.

• *Do what you can to preserve your uterus.* Hysterectomy need not be the answer, and the need for it is still hotly disputed. The removal of the uterus or the ovaries will interfere with your general well-being. Even if your tubes or ovaries are badly damaged from endometriosis, there is still no reason to regard hysterectomy as a first course of action. Childbearing, if that is your goal, may still be possible through the new fertility drugs, *in vitro* fertilization, or the GIFT method.

I hope that the information on these pages will not only benefit *your* life but the lives of others, too. I have been concentrating my interest on this disease for twenty years, and much of what I know has provided the core of this book. I hope it will encourage you to be an active partner in your health care, joining forces with a specialist who wants for you what you want for yourself. Between us all, endometriosis may never again be a health threat.

Endometriosis Specialists and Support Groups

Endometriosis has been described extensively in medical literature over the last ten years, yet there are still a great number of doctors who are not fully aware of the impact this condition can have on a woman's health if symptoms are not detected at the earliest stages so treatment can be immediately instituted. Many doctors however, have, increasingly focused their attention on endometriosis. I am pleased to provide a list of doctors across the country who I know have conducted extensive clinical research on endometriosis and who have compassionately treated women with this condition. The list is arranged alphabetically by state:

Specialists

California

Dr. Robert Israel
637 S. Lucas Ave.
Los Angeles, CA 90017
213-999-2388

Dr. Howard L. Judd
Dept. of OB/GYN
UCLA Medical Center
10833 Le Conte Ave.
Los Angeles, CA 90024
213-825-9111

Dr. Richard Marrs
1245 Wilshire Blvd.
Los Angeles, CA 90033
213-482-4552

Dr. Michael Resnick
4282 Genesee Ave., Suite 304
San Diego, CA 92117
619-278-7820

Georgia

Dr. Camran Nezhat
5555 Peachtree
Dunwoody Rd. N.E.
Atlanta, GA 30342
404-255-8778

Illinois

Dr. Donald Chatman
8111 S. Stony Island
Chicago, IL 60617
312-768-5444

Dr. W. Paul Dmowski
Dept. of OB/GYN
Rush Medical College
1753 W. Congress Pkwy.
Chicago, IL 60612
312-942-6609

Louisiana

Dr. Joseph Belina
4425 Conlin St.
Metairie, LA 70006
504-888-8494

Maine

Dr. Christiane Northrup
Women to Women
1 Pleasant St.
Yarmouth, ME 04096
207-846-6163

Dr. Joyce Vargyas
1245 Wilshire Blvd.
Los Angeles, CA 90033
213-482-4552

Dr. Louis Keith
333 S. Superior St.
Chicago, IL 60611
312-908-7532

Massachusetts

Dr. Robert Barbieri
Dept. of OB/GYN
Brigham and Women's Hospital
75 Francis St.
Boston, MA 02115
617-732-4287

New York

Dr. Michael Cummings
305 Vine St.
Liverpool, NY 13088
315-422-7201

Dr. J. Victor Reyniak
1105 Fifth Ave.
New York, NY 10028
212-410-4080

Oregon

Dr. Phillip Alberts
10373 N.E. Hancock
P.O. Box 20998
Portland, OR 97220
503-255-0918

Dr. David Redwine
Mountain View Women's Clinic
2381 N.E. Connors Ave.
Bend, OR 97701
503-382-1690

Texas

Dr. Veasy C. Buttram
7550 Fannin, Suite 104
Houston, TX 77054
713-797-9123

Self-help Organizations

Empathetic doctors may offer kind words, encouragement, and medication to help you through the more difficult times with endometriosis. Friends and family, too, may be understanding and pitch in to help you when the disease is at its most debilitating. But, I have discovered, there are moments when a sufferer needs to talk to someone who knows *firsthand* what she is going through. This need to connect to someone who shares the trials of endometriosis does not diminish efforts made in her behalf by those who care about her on a day-to-day basis. Rather, exchanging information about the disease with another woman she can identify with can not only be comforting but educational and *motivational*.

U.S.-Canadian Endometriosis Association

One woman who understood the power of such connections and how they could improve the mental and physical health of sufferers began the Endometriosis Association in 1980. Mary Lou Ballweg, a writer and victim of endometriosis herself, took the step to form such a group because she wanted answers to the baffling whys of the disease.

Headquartered in Milwaukee, Wisconsin, the Endometriosis Association has grown from a small locally based society to one that has chapters and support groups throughout the United States and Canada. Since its inception, they report, the association has helped over 100,000 sufferers while 700,000 women have received their brochures.

The association stresses the need for women with the disease to give each other support. They also recognize the importance of working with members of the medical community who can provide caring, skilled treatment for women with the disease.

What can the association do for you?

Once a member, you have access to chapters and support groups where you can meet with other women to share experiences and helpful information. Those members who don't live in an area where there are chapters or support groups can still become part of he telephone membership network, or they may call o..e of the association's crisis-call listeners. Women can also connect to one another by mail through the "Request for Contact" feature in their newsletter, which is also sent to members.

The association has compiled a list of physicians who have been recommended by its members (a number of them also appear on my introductory list). These are sympathetic doctors with an understanding of the disease and its treatment. (When you are an active member, you can request back issues of their newsletter with the feature called "The Best Doctors in Town." This should enable you to find a physician in your area.) To get more information about their services and the membership fees, call the association's toll-free telephone number: 800-992-3636. You may care to write them for information about the association or starting self-help groups at:

U.S.-Canadian Endometriosis
   Association
P.O. Box 92187
Milwaukee, WI 53202

RESOLVE, Inc.

RESOLVE, Inc., is a highly regarded self-help organization with its focus on the complications and management of infertility problems. Women with endometriosis account for about 40 percent of queries and memberships. This unique organization was started by Barbara Eck Menning, a registered nurse, who noticed there weren't any resources for women going through the crises of infertility—women who needed emotional support as well as medical referrals. Since the first time it opened its doors in Belmont, Massachusetts, in 1974, RESOLVE has grown to a national membership of over forty chapters. Over the years, their goals have remained true to the original: to help women resolve the problem of infertility. This may be through conception (after medical treatment), *in vitro* fertilization, adoption, or coming to terms with being childless.

RESOLVE offers a yearly membership, too. They publish a five-times-yearly newsletter about infertility-related issues as well as providing a medical contact system. They also run counseling services and a "geographic contact system" to help out women interested in support groups in touch with each other. National conferences and monthly events include all aspects of infertility for couples, including other options, such as adoption. To learn more about this organization and their membership rates, write to:

RESOLVE, Inc.
5 Water St.
Arlington, MA 02174
617-643-2424.

These two associations are intimately involved in the lives of women suffering from endometriosis, but there are many others that can assist you in other aspects of getting well. The list that follows includes groups that can advise you about finding a gynecologist, a laser surgeon, an expert in managing stress, and much more.

Other Self-help or Information-Gathering Associations

Biofeedback

American Association of Biofeedback Clinicians
2424 South Dempster Ave.
Des Plaines, IL 60016
312-827-0440

234

Fertility Information

The American Fertility Society
2131 Magnolia Ave.
Birmingham, AL 35205
205-251-9764

Gynecology

American College of Obstetricians and Gynecologists
600 Maryland Ave. S.W.
Washington, DC 20014
202-638-5577

Holistic Health

American Holistic Medical Association
2727 Fairview Ave. East, #D
Seattle, WA 98102
206-322-6842

International Association of Holistic Health Practitioners
3419 Thom Blvd.
Las Vegas, NV 89106
702-873-4542

Hysterectomy

Nora W. Coffey
HERS (Hysterectomy Educational Resources and Services)
501 Woodbrook Lane
Philadelphia, PA 19119
215-247-6232

Center for Climacteric Studies
University of Florida
901 N.W. Eighth Ave., Suite B-5
Gainesville, FL 32601
904-391-7172

In Vitro Fertilization/GIFT (Gamete Intrafallopian Transfer)

Dr. Elynne Margulis, Medical Director
In Vitro Fertilization/GIFT Program
Dept. of OB/GYN
Columbia Presbyterian Medical Center
622 W. 168 St.
New York, NY 10032
212-305-9921

Dr. Robert Schenken, Director
Dept. of OB/GYN
University of Texas Health Science Center
7703 Floyd Curl Dr.
San Antonio, TX 78284
512-567-4955

Dr. Richard W. Tureck, Director
In Vitro Fertilization Program
The Hospital of the University of Pennsylvania
3400 Spruce St.
Philadelphia, PA 19104
215-662-2950

(For the locations of other *in vitro* or GIFT centers, ask your doctor or contact a large medical center closest to your home.)

Laparoscopy

American Association of Gynecological Laparoscopists
11239 S. Lakewood Blvd.
Downey, CA 90241
213-862-8181

Laser Surgery

American Society for Laser Medicine and Surgery, Inc.
813 Second St., Suite 200
Wausau, WI 54401
715-845-9283

Macrobiotics

The Kushi Institute
17 Station St.
P.O. Box 1100
Brookline, MA 02147
617-738-0045

Osteoporosis

American Brittle Bone Society
1256 Merrill Dr.
Marshalton, PA 19380
215-692-6248

Pain Control

Boston Pain Center
Massachusetts Rehabilitation Hospital
125 Nashua St.
Boston, MA 02114
617-523-1818

Columbia-Presbyterian Medical Center
Pain Treatment Service
622 W. 168 St.
New York, NY 10032
212-694-7114

Duke Pain Clinic
Duke University Medical Center
Durham, NC 27710
919-684-6542

Johns Hopkins Hospital
Pain Treatment Center
Meyer Building, Room 279
Baltimore, MD 21205
301-955-3270

Mayo Clinic Pain Management Center
St. Mary's Hospital
5-D East
Rochester, MN 55902
507-284-8311

National Chronic Pain Outreach Association
822 Wycliffe Ct.
Manassas, VA 22110
703-368-8884

Rush Pain Center
Rush-Presbyterian Hospital
1725 W. Harrison St., Suite 162
Chicago, IL 60612
312-942-6631

UCLA Pain Management Center
Pelvic Pain Program
Department of Anesthesiology
UCLA School of Medicine
10833 Le Conte Ave.
Los Angeles, CA 90024
213-825-4291

University of Virginia Pain Center
University of Virginia Medical Center
Charlottesville, VA 22908
804-924-6681

(If any of these pain management centers are not conveniently located, contact a hospital or medical center in your city for the name of the center closest to you.)

Stress

Institute for Stress Management
United States International University
10455 Pomerado Rd.
San Diego, CA 92131
619-693-4753

Health Insurance Information

Insurance companies typically do not insure women who claim a "preexisting" condition when they apply for coverage, evaluating such cases as poor risks. Women with endometriosis, for example, were known to require repeated surgical procedures and to have fertility problems, incurring more than average medical expenses. Therefore, it is advisable not to state you have endometriosis until it is clinically *proved* that you have the disease. Be diagnosed and treated first.

It is my belief that contemporary women have become so much more involved in their health care that they may actually, and eventually, incur fewer expenses. Those women who are now suffering from endometriosis should not be a higher risk for something as important as health insurance. Let us hope that the approach insurance companies take toward women who are helping to cure themselves of this condition will change dramatically.

For further information about health insurance, write to:

National Insurance Consumer Organization
344 Commerce St.
Alexandria, VA 22314
703-549-8050

Group Health Association of America
Dept. NHIC
624 Ninth St. N.W., Suite 700
Washington, DC 20001
202-429-0741

Finally, be resourceful! Look into the activities offered by women's health clinics, nursing schools, health care facilities, and hospitals. If they don't have groups in progress, ask if they can refer you to an organization that can help sponsor such a network. Or start your own! You may find, as most women have who join such groups, that getting better is often as simple as helping someone else.

BIBLIOGRAPHY

"Advocates May Be Overselling Lasers for Endometriosis." *OB.GYN News.* 2/15–29/84.

"A New Approach to Chronic Pelvic Pain: An Inverview with Gay Guzinski, M.D." *The Female Patient.* 8/83.

"Asymptomatic Endometriosis Common in Infertile." *OB.GYN News.* 1987.

Barbieri, Robert L., M.D., and colleagues. "Danazol in the Treatment of Endometriosis: Analysis of 100 Cases with a 4-Year Follow-up." *Fertility and Sterility.* Vol. 37, No. 6. 6/82.

Bartosik, Delphine, M.D., and colleagues. "Endometrial Tissue in Peritoneal Fluid." *Fertility and Sterility.* Vol. 46, No. 5. 11/86.

Betts, John W., M.D., and Veasy C. Buttram, M.D. "A Plan for Managing Endometriosis." *Contemporary OB/GYN.* 4/80.

Breen, James L., M.D., and Annos, Thomas, M.D. *Differential Diagnosis in Gynecology & Obstetrics II: Endometriosis.* Ortho Pharmaceutical Corporation. 9/82.

Brody, Jane E. "Laser Lessens the Trauma of Surgery in Uterus." *The New York Times.* 4/14/87.

———. *Jane Brody's Nutrition Book.* W. W. Norton & Co. 1981.

Buttram, Veasy C., Jr., M.D. "Evolution of the Revised American Fertility Society Classification of Endometriosis." *Fertility and Sterility.* Vol. 43, No. 3. 3/85.

Buttram, Veasy C., Jr., M.D., and colleagues. "Treatment of Endometriosis with Danazol: Report of a 6-Year Prospective Study." *Fertility and Sterility.* Vol. 43, No. 3. 3/85.

Cedars, M., M.D., and colleagues. *Treatment of Endometriosis with a Long-Acting GnRH Agonist (GnRH-a) and Medroxyprogesterone Acetate (MPA).* Presented at Society for Gynecological Investigation, Thirty-fourth Annual Meeting, Atlanta, Georgia. 3/21/87.

Chatman, Donald L., M.D. "Endometriosis in the Black Woman." *American Journal of Obstetrics and Gynecology.* 8/76.

Chong, Augusto P., M.D. "Danazol Versus the Carbon Dioxide Laser Plus Postoperative Danazol." *Lasers in Surgery and Medicine,* 571–76. 1985.

Chong, Augusto P., M.D., and Michael S. Baggish. "Management of Pelvic Endometriosis by Means of Intra-abdominal Use of the Carbon Dioxide Laser." *Fertility and Sterility.* Vol. 39, No. 3. 3/83.

Chuong, C. James, M.D., and colleagues. "Vitamin B_6 Levels in Premenstrual Syndrome." Society for Gynecological Investigation, Thirty-third Annual Meeting, Toronto, Canada. 3/19/86.

Comite, F., M.D., and colleagues. *GnRH Analog Therapy in Endometriosis: Impact on Bone Mass.* Presented at Society for Gynecological Investigation, Thirty-fourth Annual Meeting, Atlanta, Georgia. 3/19/87.

Cramer, D. W., M.D., and colleagues. "Risk Factors for Endometriosis." *OB/GYN Literature News.* Vol. 6, No. 2. 1986.

Dickey, Richard P., M.D., Ph.D. *Managing Danazol Patients.* Creative Informatics, Inc. 1985.

Dizerega, Gere S., M.D., and colleagues. "Endometriosis: Role of Ovarian Steroids in Initiation, Maintenance and Suppression." *Fertility and Sterility.* 6/80.

Dmowski, W. Paul, M.D., Ph.D. "Pseudomenopause: A New Approach in Treating Endometriosis." *Contemporary OB/GYN.* Vol. 8. 8/76.

Dmowski, W. Paul, M.D., and Ewa Radwanska, M.D. "Current Concepts on Pathology, Histogenesis and Etiology of Endometriosis." *Acta Obstetrics and Gynecology Scandinavian Supplement.* 1984.

Drake, T., LCDR, M.C., U.S.N., and colleagues. "Unexplained Infertility." *Obstetrics and Gynecology.* Vol. 50, No. 6. 12/77.

Dunnett, Bill. "Drugs That Suppress Immunity." *American Health.* 11/86.

"Endometriosis Does Not Cause Infertility." *OB.GYN News.* 1986.

"Endometriosis Link to Infertility Not Explained by a Single Factor." *OB.GYN News.* 1986.

"Endometriosis Underdiagnosed, Its Rate Grossly Underestimated." *OB.GYN News.* 2/15–29/84.

Folkman, Susan, Ph.D. "Personal Control." *Journal of Personality and Social Psychology.* Vol. 46. 4/84.

Foster, Giraud V., M.D., and colleagues. "Hot Flashes in Postmenopausal Women Ameliorated by Danazol." *Fertility and Sterility.* 3/85.

Glass, Judy. "Scope Endometriosis, Zap It Away." *Medical Tribune.* 11/5/86.

Gleicher, Norbert, M.D., and colleagues. "Lymphocyte Subsets in Endometriosis." *Obstetrics & Gynecology.* Vol. 63, No. 4. 4/84.

241

Goldstein, Donald P., M.D., and colleagues. "Adolescent Endometriosis." *Journal of Adolescent Health Care.* Vol. 1, No. 1. 1980.

Greenblatt, Robert B., M.D., and Vassilious Tzingounis, M.D. "Danazol Treatment of Endometriosis: Long-term Follow-up." *Fertility and Sterility.* Vol. 32, No. 5. 11/79.

Halme, Jouko, M.D., Ph.D., and colleagues. "Retrograde Menstruation in Healthy Women and in Patients with Endometriosis." *Obstetrics & Gynecology.* Vol. 64, No. 2. 8/84.

Hammond, Charles B., M.D., and Wayne S. Maxson, M.D. "Current Status of Estrogen Replacement Therapy for the Menopause." *Fertility and Sterility.* 1/82.

Hanson, Peter G., M.D. *The Joy of Stress.* Andrews, McMeel & Parker. 1985.

Helms, Joseph M., M.D. "Acupuncture for the Management of Primary Dysmenorrhea." *Obstetrics & Gynecology.* Vol. 69, No. 1. 1/87.

Hixson, Joseph R. "LHRH Shrinks Fibroids, Delays Hysterectomies." *Medical Tribune.* 3/18/87.

"Hormone Agonists May Be Danazol Alternative in Endometriosis." *OB.GYN News.* 7/15–31/85.

Hull, Magdalen E., M.D., and Colleagues. "Comparison of Different Modalities of Endometriosis in Infertile Women." *Fertility and Sterility.* Vol. 47, No. 1. 1/87.

"Immunology Plays Important Role in Endometriosis, Studies Suggest." *OB.GYN News.* 2/15–29/84.

Janne, O., M.D., and colleagues. "Estrogen and Progestin Receptors in Endometriotic Lesions: Comparison with Endometriotic Tissue." *American Journal of Obstetrics and Gynecology.* 11/81.

Jenkins, Susan, M.D., and colleagues. "Endometriosis: Pathogenic Implications of the Anatomic Distribution." *Obstetrics & Gynecology.* Vol. 67, No. 3. 3/86.

Johnson, William M., III, M.D., and Charles M. Tyndal, M.D. "Pulmonary Endometriosis: Treatment with Danazol." *Obstetrics and Gynecology.* Vol. 69, No. 3. 3/87.

Jones, G. S., M.D., and colleagues. "The Role of Pituitary Gonadotropins in Follicular Stimulation and Oocyte Maturation in the Human." *Journal of Clinical Endocrinology and Metabolism.* Vol. 59, No. 1. 1984.

Kadar, Peter, C.A. "An Oriental Approach to Sexual Dysfunction." *Whole Life Times.* 10/86.

Karnaky, Karl John, M.D. "The Effect of Stilboestrol on the Formed Elements of the Blood in Women." *Journal of Obstetrics and Gynecology.* Vol. 54, No. 3. 6/47.

Karnes, Diane. "How Nutrition Helped My Gynecological Problems." *Prevention.* 8/79.

Kauppila, Antti, M.D., and colleagues. "Effect of Gestrinone in Endometriosis Tissue and Endometrium." *Fertility and Sterility.* Vol. 44, No. 4. 10/85.

Keye, W. R., Jr., M.D., and colleagues. "Feasibility Studies of the Argon Laser in the Treatment of Endometriosis." *Fertility and Sterility.* Vol. 39, No. 3. 3/83.

Khan-Dawood, Firyal S., M.D., and colleagues. *Peritoneal Fluid Estrogen, Progesterone, Gonadotropins and Prolactin in Normal Women and in Women with Endometriosis.* Presented at Society for Gynecological Investigation, Thirty-third Annual Meeting, Toronto, Canada. 3/19/86.

Kistner, Robert W., M.D., and colleagues. "Suggested Classification for Endometriosis: Relationship to Endometriosis." Abstract Supplement, *Fertility and Sterility.* 3/77.

Kistner, Robert W., M.D., and Robert Barbieri, M.D. "Endometriosis." Chapter Nine in *Gynecology: Principles and Practice.* Boston: Harvard Medical School. 1986.

Kornfield, Donald S., M.D. "Psychological Considerations in Management of Pain—Part 2." *Physician and Patient.* 6/85.

Lamb, Karen, R.N., Ph.D., and Nancy Berg, B.A. "Tampon Use in Women with Endometriosis." *Journal of Community Health.* Vol. 10, No. 4. Winter 1985.

Lamb, Karen, R.N., Ph.D., and colleagues. "Family Trait Analysis: A Case Control Study of 43 Women with Endometriosis and Their Best Friends." *American Journal of Obstetrics and Gynecology.* 3/86.

"Laser Held Effective in Infertility of Endometriosis." *OB.GYN News.* 2/1–14/86.

"Laser Shopping: All Are Not Created Equal." *Medical Tribune.* 11/5/86.

Lauersen, Niels H., M.D., and Eileen Stukane. *Listen to Your Body.* Fireside/Simon & Schuster. 1982.

Lauersen, Niels H., M.D., and Kathleen H. Wilson, B.S. "The Effect of Danazol in the Treatment of Chronic Cystic Mastitis." *Obstetrics & Gynecology.* Vol. 48, No. 1. 7/76.

———. "Evaluation of Danazol as an Oral Contraceptive." *Obstetrics and Gynecology.* Vol. 50, No. 1. 7/77.

Lauersen, Niels H., M.D., and colleagues. "Danazol: An Antigonadal Agent in the Treatment of Endometriosis." *American Journal of Obstetrics and Gynecology.* 12/75.

LeMay, André, M.D., Ph.D., and colleagues. "Reversible Hypogonadism Induced by a Luteinizing Hormone-Releasing Hormone (LH-RH) Agonist (Buserelin) as a New Therapeutic Approach for Endometriosis." *Fertility and Sterility.* Vol. 41, No. 6. 6/84.

Longo, Lawrence D., M.D. "Classic Pages in Obstetrics and Gynecology: Experimental Endometriosis." *American Journal of Obstetrics and Gynecology.* 8/78.

"Luck, Therapy in Endometriosis Help Preserve Fertility of Teen." *OB.GYN News.* Vol. 17, No. 18.

Malinak, L. Russell, M.D. "Pelvic Pain—When Is Surgery Indicated?" *Contemporary OB/GYN.* 8/85.

Malinak, L. Russell, M.D., and colleagues. "Heritable Aspects of Endometriosis II: Clinical Characteristics of Familial Endometriosis." *American Journal of Obstetrics and Gynecology.* 6/80.

"Managing Infertile Patient with Mild Endometriosis." *OB.GYN News.* 1986.

Marrs, Richard P., M.D., and Joyce M. Vargyas, M.D. "Pelvic Endometriosis." Chapter 29 of *Infertility, Contraception and Reproductive Endocrinology.* 2d ed. 1986.

Mastroianni, Luigi, M.D., and Tureck, Richard W., M.D. "The Challenge of Pelvic Endometriosis: A Dialogue with Case Histories." *OBGdiagnosis.* Vol. 1, Iss. 2. 1983.

Meigs, Joe Vincent, M.D. *The Medical Treatment of Endometriosis and the Significance of Endometriosis.* Presented at Clinical Congress of the American College of Surgeons. 10/48.

Mercaitis, Patricia, Ph.D., and colleagues. "Effect of Danazol on Vocal Pitch: A Case Study. *Obstetrics & Gynecology.* Vol. 65, No. 1. 1/85.

"Mild Endometriosis Tied to Spontaneous Abortions." *OB.GYN News.* 1987.

Muscato, Joseph J., M.D., and colleagues. "Sperm Phagocytosis by Human Peritoneal Macrophages: A Possible Cause of Infertility in Endometriosis." *American Journal of Obstetrics and Gynecology.* 1982.

Muse, Ken N., M.D., and Emery A. Wilson, M.D. "How Does Mild Endometriosis Cause Infertility?" *Fertility and Sterility.* Vol. 38, No. 2. 8/82.

Nezhat, Camran, M.D., and colleagues. "Videolaseroscopy for the Treatment of Endometriosis and Other Diseases of the Reproductive Organs." *Obstetrics and Gynecology Forum.* Vol. 1. Jan./Feb. 1987.

Parachini, Allan. "A New Endometriosis Treatment." *The Los Angeles Times.* 5/27/86.

Parsons, Anna K., M.D., and colleagues. *Buserelin Versus Danazol Therapy of Endometriosis: Pituitary Hormone and Estrogen Changes.* Presented at Society for Gynecological Investigation, Thirty-fourth Annual Meeting, Atlanta, Georgia. 3/20/87.

Patton, Phillip E., M.D., and colleagues. "CA-125 Levels in Endometriosis." *Fertility and Sterility.* Vol. 45, No. 6. 6/86.

Pearson, Durk, and Sandy Shaw. *Life Extension: A Practical Scientific Approach.* Warner Books. 1982.

Pittaway, Donald E., M.D., Ph.D., and Wentz, Anne C., M.D. "Endometriosis and Corpus Luteum Function." *Journal of Reproductive Medicine.* Vol. 29, No. 10. 10/84.

Pittaway, Donald E., M.D., and colleagues. "Luteal Phase Defects in Infertility Patients with Endometriosis." *Fertility and Sterility.* 10/83.

"Presence of 'Pepper Spots' Warrants a Dx of Endometriosis." *OB.GYN News.* 1987.

Randal, Judith. "Nostrums for Cramps." *Newsday.* 1985.

Restak, Richard, M.D. *The Brain.* Bantam Books. 1984.

Reyniak, J. Victor, M.D., and Niels H. Lauersen, M.D. "Danazol—a Versatile Pharmacologic Agent." *Fertility and Sterility.* Vol. 37, No. 4. 4/82.

Rothberg, Lee. "Hysterectomy: The Shocking Truth." *Woman's Newspaper.* Iss. 54. 9/86.

Sampson, John A., M.D. "Peritoneal Endometriosis Due to the Menstrual Dissemination of Endometrial Tissue into the Peritoneal Cavity." *American Journal of Obstetrics and Gynecology.* 1927.

Schenken, Robert S., M.D., and colleagues. *Effect of Pregnancy on Endometriosis in Cynomologus Monkeys.* Presented at Society for Gynecologic Investigation, Thirty-fourth Annual Meeting, Atlanta, Georgia. 3/19/87.

Schmeck, Harold M., Jr. "Burst of Discoveries Reveals Genetic Basis for Many Diseases." *The New York Times.* 3/31/87.

"Secondary Sex Ratio Altered in Births After Mild Endometriosis." *OB.GYN News.* 1987.

Seibel, Machelle, M.D., and colleagues. "The Effectiveness of Danazol on Subsequent Fertility in Minimal Endometriosis." *Fertility and Sterility.* Vol. 38, No. 5. 11/82.

Shamsudden, A.K.M., M.D., and colleagues. "Adenocarcinoma Arising from Extragonadal Endometriosis 14 Years After Total Hysterectomy and Bilateral Salpingo-oophorectomy for Endometriosis." *American Journal of Obstetrics and Gynecology.* 3/79.

Simpson, Joe Leigh, M.D., and colleagues. "Heritable Aspects of Endometriosis I: Genetic Studies." *American Journal of Obstetrics and Gynecology.* 6/80.

Steele, Russell W., M.D., and colleagues. "Immunologic Aspects of Human Endometriosis." *American Journal of Reproductive Immunology.* 3/84.

Steingold, K. A., M.D., and colleagues. "Treatment of Endometriosis with a Long-Acting Gonadotropin-Releasing Hormone Agonist." *Obstetrics & Gynecology.* Vol. 69, No. 3. 3/87.

"Still No Gold Standard for Infertile with Endometriosis." *OB.GYN News.* 1/1–14/85.

Thompson, Suzanne C., Ph.D. "Control and Stress." *Psychological Bulletin.* 7/81.

Trubo, Richard. "Stress and Disease: Cellular Evidence Hints at Therapy." *Medical World News.* 1/29/87.

Tureck, Richard W., M.D. "Laser Laparoscopy: Lesions Go Up in Smoke." *Masters in Obstetrics and Gynecology.* Vol. 2, No. 2. Fall 1986.

"Ultrasonography Neither Sensitive, Specific in Dx of Endometriosis." *OB.GYN News.* Vol. 21, No. 1. 1987.

Vernon, Michael W., Ph.D., and colleagues. "Classification of Endometriotic Implants by Morphological Appearance and Capacity to Synthesize Prostaglandins. *Fertility and Sterility.* Vol. 46, No. 5. 11/86.

Vernon, Michael W., Ph.D., and colleagues. "Human Chorionic Gonadotropin (hCG) Suppresses Endometriosis in the Rat Model." Presented at Society for Gynecological Investigation. 3/21/87.

Weiss, Gerson, M.D., ed. *Endometriosis: Approach to Management. Proceedings of the Endometriosis Symposium.* NYU Post-Graduate Medical School, Winthrop Pharmaceuticals. 10/85.

Wheeler, James M., M.D., and colleagues. "The Relationship of Endometriosis to Spontaneous Abortion." *Fertility and Sterility.* 5/83.

Wilson, Emery A., M.D., ed. *Endometriosis.* Alan R. Liss, Inc. 1987.

Ylikorkala, Olavi, M.D., and colleagues. "Peritoneal Fluid Prostaglandins in Endometriosis, Tubal Disorders and Unexplained Infertility." *Obstetrics & Gynecology.* Vol. 63, No. 5. 5/84.

INDEX

247

About the Authors

NIELS H. LAUERSEN, M.D., Ph.D., is Clinical Professor of Obstetrics and Gynecology at New York Medical College and is in private practice in New York City. More than 1 million copies of his five highly regarded books for the general public (including *PMS: Premenstrual Syndrome and You, Listen to Your Body*, and *It's Your Pregnancy*) have been sold. He has appeared on the "Phil Donahue Show," "Good Morning America," "Hour Magazine," "Sonya" and elsewhere, contributes regularly to *Cosmopolitan*, and has been featured in *Vogue, Harper's Bazaar, Working Woman*, and other publications. His three textbooks and more than eighty scholarly articles have earned him international recognition.

Writer CONSTANCE DESWAAN has collaborated with Dr. Sonya Friedman on her three best-selling books, and has written numerous other business and health-related books. Her articles have appeared in major magazines. She lives in New York City.